Behaviors and Persistence of Nanomaterials in Biomedical Applications

Scrivener Publishing
100 Cummings Center, Suite 541J
Beverly, MA 01915-6106

Advances in Nanotechnology & Applications

Series Editor: Madhuri Sharon

The unique properties of nanomaterials encourage the belief that they can be applied in a wide range of fields, from medical applications to electronics, environmental sciences, information and communication, heavy industries like aerospace, refineries, automobile, consumer and sports good, etc.

This book series will focus on the properties and related applications of nanomaterials so as to have a clear fundamental picture as to why nanoparticles are being tried instead of traditional methods. Since nanotechnology is encompassing various fields of science, each book will focus on one topic and will detail the basics to advanced science for the benefit of all levels of researchers.

Series Editor: Madhuri Sharon, Director, Walchand Centre for Research in Nanotechnology & Bionanotechnology
W.H. Marg, Ashok Chowk, Solapur 413 006
Maharashtra,
India

E-mail:sharonmadhuri@gmail.com

Publishers at Scrivener
Martin Scrivener (martin@scrivenerpublishing.com)
Phillip Carmical (pcarmical@scrivenerpublishing.com)

Behaviors and Persistence of Nanomaterials in Biomedical Applications

Domenico Cassano
and Valerio Voliani

Scrivener Publishing

WILEY

This edition first published 2018 by John Wiley & Sons, Inc., 111 River Street, Hoboken, NJ 07030, USA and Scrivener Publishing LLC, 100 Cummings Center, Suite 541J, Beverly, MA 01915, USA

For more information about Scrivener publications please visit www.scrivenerpublishing.com.

Wiley Global Headquarters
111 River Street, Hoboken, NJ 07030, USA

For details of our global editorial offices, customer services, and more information about Wiley products visit us at www.wiley.com.

Library of Congress Cataloging-in-Publication Data

ISBN 978-1-119-41827-6

Cover image: Pixabay.Com
Cover design by Russell Richardson

Set in size of 13pt and Minion Pro by Exeter Premedia Services Private Ltd., Chennai, India

10 9 8 7 6 5 4 3 2 1

Contents

Preface

Nanomaterials have demonstrated the potential to revolutionize the way in which neoplasms are diagnosed and treated. Some efficient treatments relying on organic nanomaterials are already on the market, while even more promising ones based on noble metals are still at the bench level. Organism persistence after medical action is a major concern hampering the clinical translation of metal nanoparticles. Today, the most practical way to avoid undesirable toxic effects, while maintaining desirable imaging/therapeutic moieties, is by engineering all-in-one biodegradable nanoplatforms that are excretable through the renal pathway after the designed medical action. Despite the field being very young, in the near future personalized and effective treatments of neoplasms may no longer be a dream but a real possibility. The potentiality of these novel nanotheranostics is impressive, but a lot of work is yet to be done.

In order to introduce you to the "world of nanomaterials," the scope of this book is outlined in Chapter 1 and a comprehensive review of the behaviors of both organic and inorganic nanomaterials is presented in Chapter 2. In Chapter 3, the promising applications in diagnosis and treatment of neoplasms are discussed. The interactions of nanomaterials with biological systems at both the cellular and body levels are presented in Chapter 4, together with the main drawback of metal nanomaterials—the issue of persistence. In Chapter 5, the actual FDA and EMA approval pipeline for nanotheranostics and the nanomaterials that have reached the market are introduced. Chapter 6 reports the most advanced and promising approaches for avoiding the issue of persistence. Finally, in Chapter 7, along with conclusions drawn from the material presented, the perspectives of this exciting fields are discussed.

This book offers state-of-the-art and comprehensive coverage of nanomaterials ranging from their behaviors to the market. In particular, the issue of persistence is discussed, and the most promising approaches to unlock the potentiality of metal nanomaterials for innovative noninvasive and efficient treatments of neoplasms are presented. General readers of this book will gain complete insight into nanomaterials, physicians will have a guide to the latest information on the novel tools under development, and biologists/chemists/physicists/engineers will have a guide for designing the next generation of nanotheranostics.

Domenico Cassano and Valerio Voliani
Pisa, Italy
March 2018

1

Introduction

Industry analysts have been forecasting groundbreaking advances as a result of nanotechnology application in renewable energy, communications, pollution removals, agriculture, and medicine [1]. Clothing, sunscreens, cosmetics, sporting equipment, batteries, food packaging, dietary supplements, and electronics are just a few of the kinds of nanotechnology-enabled goods in use [1]. For example, nanosized: i) silver is used in food packaging, ii) silica is employed in food additives, and iii) titanium dioxide, gold, platinum, and zinc oxide are used in cosmetics, such as sunscreens and toothpastes [2, 3]. Although there are several uses of nanomaterials in daily products, the most promising application is in the medical field [2]. A lot of excitement has been generated during last decades about the medical and economic impact of nano-technological approaches in healthcare [4]. The first medical nanosystem was introduced in human therapy at the end of the last century to increase the efficacy of known, but poorly bioavailable drugs [5]. Today, research on nanomaterials is aimed to decrease the side-effects of therapies while increase their action thanks to the unique physical, chemical and physiological features of the matter at the nanoscale. Such advances include improved early screening and diagnosis, as well as treatment regimens that have reduced off-target toxicity; areas where nanoparticle approach is likely to have significant future impact [6].

The usual target application of nanomaterials is related to diagnosis and therapy of neoplasms, due to a number of key-properties of nanomaterials. These behaviors include size, payload density, duration of effect, and surface properties/targeting [6]. For example, the pharmacokinetic profile of nanoparticle-incorporated drugs often includes a dramatic increase in circulation half-life ($t_{1/2}$) compared to the drug alone [6]. Moreover, nanoparticles show the possibility to insert many functionalities on the same platform in order to develop "multifunctional" nanoparticles (theranostic agents) able to improve delivery, therapeutic efficacy, and ultimately patient outcome [7]. Theranostic agents can simultaneously deliver imaging and therapeutic actions to specific sites or organs, enabling detection and treatment of disease in a single procedure [7].

Nanomaterials can be divided in two class: soft and hard [8]. The first are composed by polymers, lipid vesicles and polymer-protein conjugates, while the latter are based on inorganic materials, and in particular metals. Noble metals, due to the high atomic number and the Localized Plasmon Surface Resonances (LSPRs), intrinsically possess both imaging and therapeutic capabilities. This results in more profound benefits in the design of theranostics, holding the great promise to shift current medical detection and therapy paradigms [9].

To date, more than 40 nanosystems for healthcare applications are in the market. The large majority of these nanosystems are soft nanomaterials [5]. Just four metal-based nanomaterials (iron oxide) are already in the market, following the 1996 approval of Endorem® (Guerbet) by the FDA for Magnetic Resonance Imaging (MRI) diagnostics [8]. Remarkably, there is still no approved nanomaterials based on noble metals for cancer therapy [5, 8]. The only approved platform using gold nanosphere is a tool for bench diagnostic [5]. The lack of translation of metal nanoparticles to the market is mainly related to the concern of their persistence in organisms after the action, confining all their intriguing feature to the bench-side [8]. Recently, nanomaterials designed by the ultrasmall-in-nano approach able to jointly combine theranostic applications and metal excretion were proposed, holding the promise to unlock the appealing behaviors of metal nanomaterials for groundbreaking cancer treatments.

The purpose of this Volume is to collect and comprehensively discuss the advances in this current and exciting topic in order to promote and enhance its growth. In the first part of the Volume, a general introduction about the main features of both organic and inorganic nanomaterials is provided. Then, the most promising and innovative applications for cancer treatment and diagnostic are introduced.

In the second part, an analysis of the nanomaterials in the market for healthcare applications is presented. The issue of unwanted accumulation of metals in organisms after the designed action is then discussed. Finally, the most recent progresses in the design of nanomaterials that are able to escape from organisms after the selected action are comprehensively described, and the perspectives of this exciting field provided.

This Volume is intended for academics at every stage of career and to professionals interested in nanomaterials.

References

1. Kessler, R. Engineered Nanoparticles in Consumer Products: Understanding a New Ingredient. *Environ. Health Perspect.* 119, a120–a125, 2011.

2. Fröhlich, E. & Roblegg, E. Models for oral uptake of nanoparticles in consumer products. *Toxicology* 291, 10–17, 2012.
3. Love, S. a, Maurer-Jones, M. a, Thompson, J. W., Lin, Y.-S. & Haynes, C. L. Assessing nanoparticle toxicity. *Annu. Rev. Anal. Chem.* 5, 181–205, 2012.
4. Schütz, C. A., Juillerat-Jeanneret, L., Soltmann, C. & Mueller, H. Toxicity data of therapeutic nanoparticles in patent documents. *World Pat. Inf.* 35, 110–114, 2013.
5. Schütz, C. a, Juillerat-Jeanneret, L., Mueller, H., Lynch, I. & Riediker, M. Therapeutic nanoparticles in clinics and under clinical evaluation. *Nanomedicine* 8, 449–467, 2013.
6. Heidel, J. D. & Davis, M. E. Clinical developments in nanotechnology for cancer therapy. *Pharm. Res.* 28, 187–199, 2011.
7. Cheng, Z., Al Zaki, A., Hui, J. Z., Muzykantov, V. R. & Tsourkas, A. Multifunctional Nanoparticles: Cost Versus Benefit of Adding Targeting and Imaging Capabilities. *Science (80-.).* 338, 903–910, 2012.
8. Etheridge, M. L. *et al.* The big picture on nanomedicine: The state of investigational and approved nanomedicine products. *Nanomedicine Nanotechnology, Biol. Med.* 9, 1–14, 2013.
9. Yu, M. & Zheng, J. Clearance Pathways and Tumor Targeting of Imaging Nanoparticles. *ACS Nano* 9 (7), pp 6655–6674, 2015.

2

Nanomaterials

The behaviors of matter at the nanoscale are fascinating and completely different with respect to the bulk. In this chapter, we address this topic: in the first part, the intriguing and unexpected behavior of materials at the nanoscale are presented, while in the second part, an overview of the most popular nanomaterials and their general method of production is provided, focusing on wet chemical synthesis routes.

2.1 Physical Properties of Nanomaterials

Science and technology have been deeply revolutionized over the past decades, since when the controlled production of materials in the size range of 1–100 nm (referred to as nanomaterials) has been improved. Because of the small size, most of the physical, physiological and chemical properties of materials at the nanoscale are completely different from those of the bulk.

Indeed, within this size-range, features such as melting point, hardness, optical behavior, catalytic activity, or magnetic permeability become size-dependent. These peculiar behaviors are also ascribed to the surface-to-volume ratio, which decreases proportionally to the inverse particle size. A strictly related quantity is the dispersion, which is defined as ratio between the surface atoms and the total number of atoms (N) and scale as $N^{1/3}$.

A more rigorous interpretation is related to the number of direct atom's neighbors, or coordination number. Considering a crystal lattice, it is easy to Figure that atoms at the surface, edges and corners, have fewer neighbors and are weakly bound than those in the bulk. Considering a cubic lattice, an atom in the core has 6 direct neighbors while at the interface has 5 direct neighbors (Figure 2.1). Proceeding from the core towards the surface, atoms will lower their coordination since at the edge they will have 4 direct neighbors and only 3 at the corners. This is why the surface has a higher energy and many of the properties of the materials are surface-dependent (*e.g.*, melting starts from the surface, not from the core) [1].

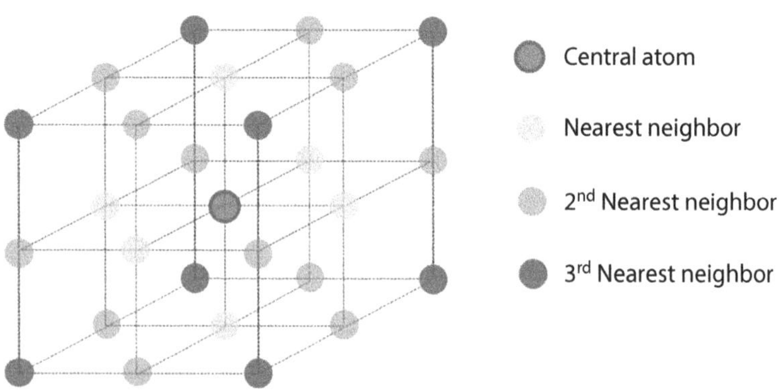

Figure 2.1 Portion of a three-dimensional cubic crystal lattice. First, second and third nearest neighbors, with respect to the central atom, are marked with different gray levels.

Next, we briefly review some of the physical properties of materials at the nanoscale, also suggesting some significant theoretical details.

2.1.1 Thermodynamic Properties: Melting Point Depression and Superheating

In bulk materials, thermodynamic properties are investigated as macroscopic ensembles of particles, in which only the most probable distribution is taken into account and it is subjected to classical Boltzmann or quantum Fermi-Dirac and Bose-Einstein statistics, depending on the physical conditions. In those macroscopic systems, thermodynamic quantities such as local temperature are well defined, even though fluctuations exist, because they can be considered stable as they scale with the inverse square root of the number of particles, which are of the order of the Avogadro number N_A. When the systems are reduced to nanometer size, it is not easy to define temperature since N is by far smaller than in the bulk, and fluctuations become of the same order of magnitude of the thermodynamic quantities, which varies randomly and unpredictably over time.

This behavior has deep implications in all the thermodynamic properties of materials, such as the melting point of solids. Phase transitions, indeed, are collective phenomena in which there is a sharp temperature at which a phase is lost because all the atoms interact differently in different phases. Due to the number of atoms related to the nanosized regime, the phase transitions are no more so sharp. Indeed, a number of phases can coexist at the same temperature as shown in Figure 2.2.

In particular, two phenomena are strongly affected in the nanosized regime: melting point, and superheating. According to Lindemann empirical criterion, melting of solids occurs when lattice vibration due to increased temperature is so high that it leads to collision between neighboring atoms, destabilizing the solid phase [3]. Lindemann criterion was reformulated in a more rigorous form by Gilvarry, according to which the

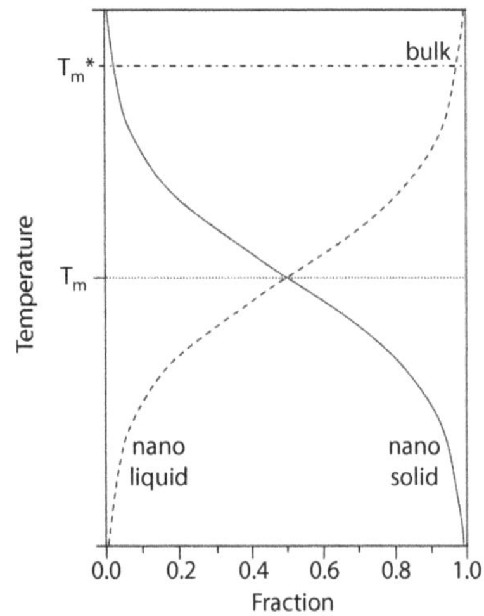

Figure 2.2 Solid/liquid phase diagram for bulk (dash-dotted straight line) and nano materials (solid and dashed curves) [2].

melting occurs when the root mean square amplitude of lattice vibration reaches a critical value which is a fraction of the spacing between nearest neighbors [4].

This criterion is a key point in understanding the phenomenon of melting point depression at the nanoscale, *i.e.* the lower melting temperature of solids in the nanosized regime with respect to bulk. Atoms on the surface interacts weakly with neighbors with respect to the ones in the core, because of lower coordination, hence, less energy has to be supplied to them to reach the critical vibration. Thus, melting of solids begins from the surface edges and proceeds towards lattice interior. It is worth to notice that surface to volume ratio in nanomaterials is much higher than in the bulk, resulting in an enhancement in the surface dependent physical features. For instance, Figure 2.3 shows melting point depression effect for Sn nanoparticles (NPs) of increasing radius, ranging from 5 to 50 nm 500Å.

Another important size-dependent thermodynamic property is related to the range of temperatures at which melting occurs. Indeed, it undergoes to a substantial broadening, which

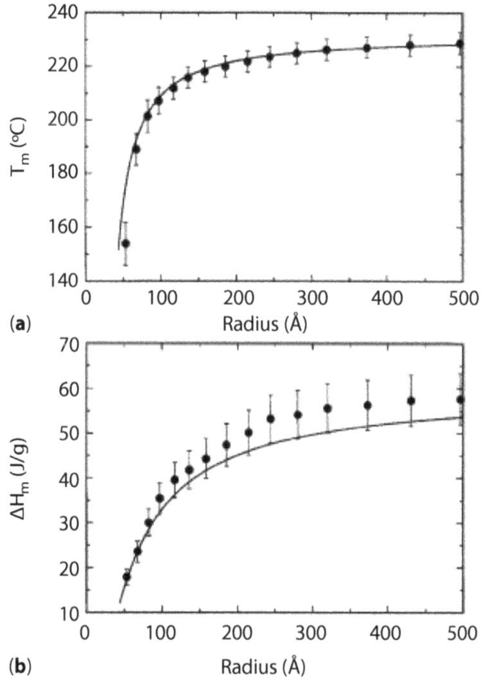

Figure 2.3 Melting temperatures (top) and heat of fusion (down) vs particle radius for Sn NPs [5]. Reprinted with permission from [5]. Copyright 1996 by the American Physical Society.

is more pronounced in smaller particles. However, there is a critical size at which surface and core cannot be distinguished anymore, thus, in ultrasmall nanoparticle regime (below 2 nm), melting occurs at a well-defined temperature, with a sharp phase transition as for the bulk [6].

Embedded NPs can show different thermodynamic behaviors in relation to the matrix in which are embedded (surface coating). For example, superheating phenomenon can be observed on coated NPs, in which melting temperature is increased if compared to bare NPs. This is related to some coatings that can somehow impair surface melting, shifting phase transition to temperatures which can be even higher than in the bulky state.

However, experimental observation of superheating is not an easy task. Some strategies involved the heating of the core while keeping the surface at lower temperature, or the stabilization of the surface edges, by coating them with materials which possess higher melting temperature with respect to the core and impairing heat diffusion at the particle/matrix interface. The second strategy is the easiest and, thus, the most used to provide experimental proof of superheating [7].

Superheating of silver NPs was observed by Daeges *et al.* by a thermal insulation approach [8]. They have coated Ag NPs with a gold shell which served as surface melting suppressor, obtaining an increase in melting temperature of 25 K. However, surface melting suppression can be also achieved by impairing surface atoms vibrations through the growth of an epitaxial layer on the NPs. The most significant examples are Pb and In nanocrystals in aluminum embedding matrix, which were observed to suffer from melting depression or superheating depending on the epitaxy matrix [9, 10]. As a general concept, these results were explained physically with an inversion in the melting propagation: melting starts from the core and proceeds towards the surface for embedded NPs, while starting from the surface and proceeds inwards for bare NPs.

2.1.2 Optical Properties

Metals

Light interacts with matter in a number of ways. When white light interacts with an object, it can be either partially or completely absorbed, reflected or transmitted. The origin of the colors we address to materials is due to the energy of the photons which strikes back from the irradiated matter to our eyes. For example, many metals have a silvery color because they have a strong reflectivity on the entire visible spectrum, while gold appears yellow because it has low reflectivity at short wavelengths. At the nanoscale, the color of metals is not as easily predictable as in the bulk.

Indeed, when the size of certain noble metals is reduced to the nanoscale, a strong peculiar interaction with light in the visible region of the electromagnetic spectrum is encountered.

This interaction depends on the size, the shape and the external medium by which metal NPs are surrounded. This optical phenomenon is attributed to collective conduction band electron oscillation in response to the electrical field of the interacting light on NPs, and is known as Localized Surface Plasmon Resonance (LSPR). For the most investigated metals in the nano-range, *i.e.* silver and gold, almost any color, from UV to near infrared (NIR), can be produced by simply controlling the shape and size of the particle [11].

LSPR can be explained by the Drude model. This theoretical model simplifies electrical conduction in metals by considering electrons as a free non-interacting gas that randomly moves in a lattice made of oppositely charged massive ions. When the action of an electric field imposes the displacement of electrons from their rest position, they begin to oscillate around the equilibrium position at a plasma frequency, $\omega_{p,}$ which is a function of the electron mass and density. The phase lag of electrons with respect to the electric field is described by the imaginary component of the dielectric function $\varepsilon(\omega) = \varepsilon_1 + i\varepsilon_2$, which fully describes the macroscopic electronic response of the material. In the Drude model, plasma frequency and dielectric function are related as $\varepsilon D(\omega) = 1 - \omega^2_p/\omega(\omega + i/\tau)$ where τ is the scattering time and encompasses all electron scattering.

For spherical NPs of volume V, interacting with electromagnetic radiation of wavelength λ_0, in a medium of dielectric constant ε_m, Maxwell's equations can be analytically solved by Mie theory in the dipole approximation, providing light scattering and absorption cross sections σ:

$$\sigma_{sca} = \frac{24\pi^3 V^2 s_m^2}{\lambda_0^4} \frac{\left(s_1 - s_m\right)^2 + s_2^2}{\left(s_1 + 2s_m\right)^2 + s_2^2} \tag{1}$$

$$\sigma_{abs} = \frac{18\pi V s_m^{\frac{3}{2}}}{\lambda_0} \frac{s_2}{\left(s_1 + 2s_m\right)^2 + s_2^2} \tag{2}$$

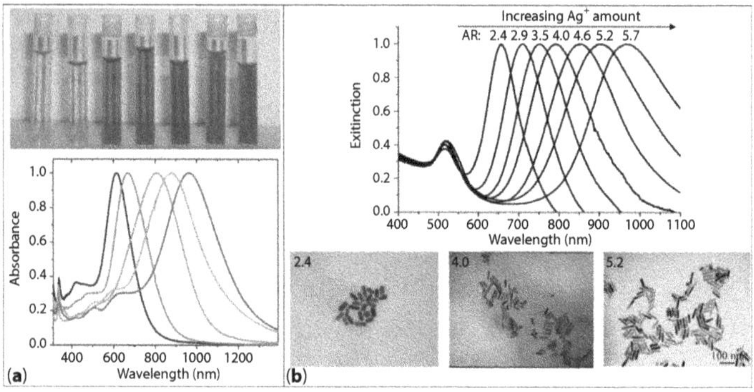

Figure 2.4 Silver (a) and gold (b) nanostructures with plasmonic response finely tunable in the UV/NIR range [13, 14]. a) is reproduced from [13] with permission of The Royal Society of Chemistry. b) is reproduced from [14] with permession of John Wiley & Sons Inc.

which provides the condition at which a resonance is excited, *i.e.* when $\varepsilon_1 = 2\varepsilon_m$ for small ε_2. LSPRs can be tuned over the entire visible electromagnetic spectrum, from UV to NIR, by tuning size, shape and environment of noble metals at the nanoscale [12]. An example is shown in Figure 2.4, where a fine tuning of plasmon resonance over a wide range of wavelengths is obtained for both silver and gold nanostructures.

The extinction of light by nanospheres (equations 1 and 2), scales with V for absorption and V^2 for scattering. Thus, the absorption effects increase by decreasing the NPs size. By further size reduction, the diameter of metal NPs dwindles down to few nanometers or even to sub-nanometer region (clusters). Clusters are composed by few atoms (less than 500) and their size is usually estimated by the element-specific Wigner-Seitz approach [15]. In the clusters regime, physical properties cannot be described anymore by bulk-like electron models, but at a molecular-like level. Thus, discrete energy levels and HOMO-LUMO gaps must be taken into account, giving rise to the loss of LSPRs and the appearance of peculiar photoluminescence in the visible to NIR region.

Clusters have become interesting sensing and imaging materials due to their long lifetime, large Stokes shift, and biocompatibility. Moreover, the photoluminescence can be finely tuned over a huge range of wavelength, as shown in Figure 2.5.

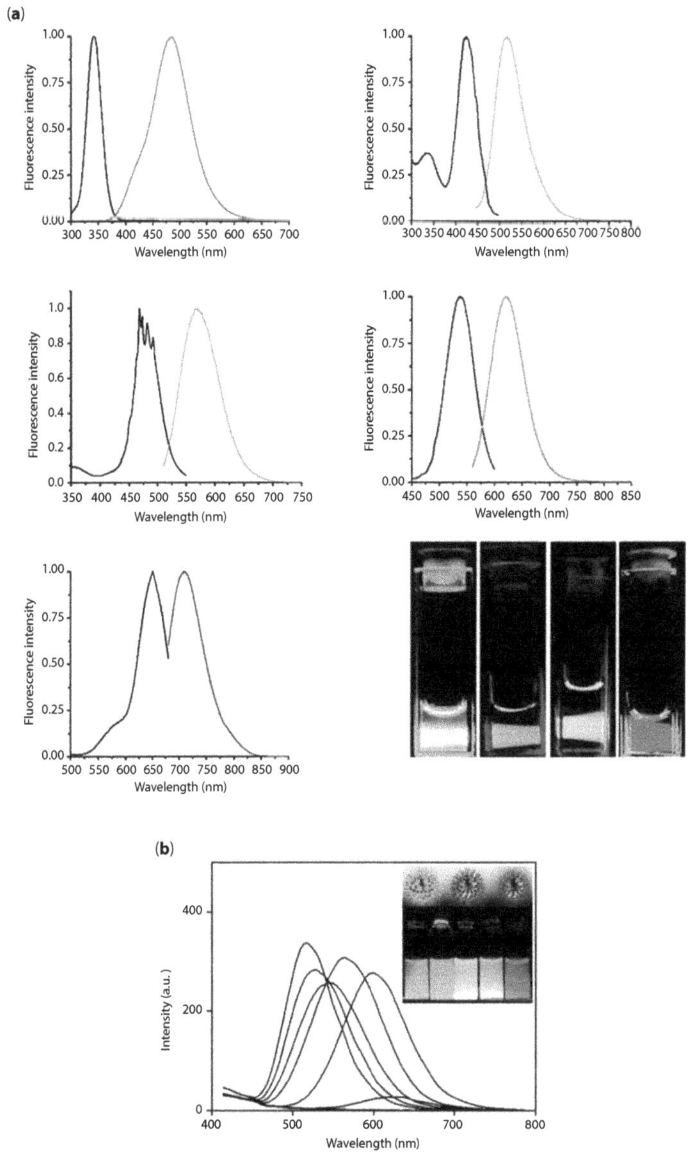

Figure 2.5 Excitation and emission spectra of Ag clusters (a) and Au clusters (b) with emission tunable over a wide range of visible wavelengths. [16, 17]. a) is reproduced from with permission from [16]. Copyright 2008 American Chemical Society. b) is reproduced from [17] with permission of the Royal Society of Chemistry.

Semiconductors

Optical properties of semiconductors are governed by transitions of electrons from valence to conduction bands, creating electron-hole pairs known as excitons. After the recombination, the exciton's energy can be emitted by radiative decay as luminescence, with a wavelength related to the energy gap between the two bands. In bulk semiconductors, the band gap energies are in the range from 0.17 eV to 3.6 eV at 300K, related to their composition and temperature [18]. The size of the semiconductor does not affect the band gap energy until the electrons are delocalized over the entire semiconductor, because no quantum effect occurs. When at least one of the dimension is small enough to produce quantum confinement (*i.e.*, when one of the dimension is comparable to the electrons coherence length), discrete energy levels in an atomic-like fashion appears. In analogy with quantum wells, the gap between the highest energy valence level and the lower energy conduction level increases with increasing confinement.

Quantum confined semiconductor nanomaterials are called quantum dots (QDs). Their absorption and emission, oppositely to bulk, is easily tunable by reducing or increasing the size of the particle. A decrease in the size causes a blue shift of the emission, whereas an increase produces a red shift. Size-dependent absorption of semiconductor quantum dots is thus extremely finely tunable and one can ideally design any wavelength-specific luminescent nanoparticle [19]. Figure 2.6 shows electron microscopy images and photoluminescence (PL) of PbSe quantum dots, whose wavelength is finely tunable in the mid-infrared region by varying their size [20].

2.1.3 Magnetism

Magnetism, in an extremely simplified picture, is produced by electrons, which bear an intrinsic spin moment (S) and the so-called orbital moment (L) produced by their electrical charge in

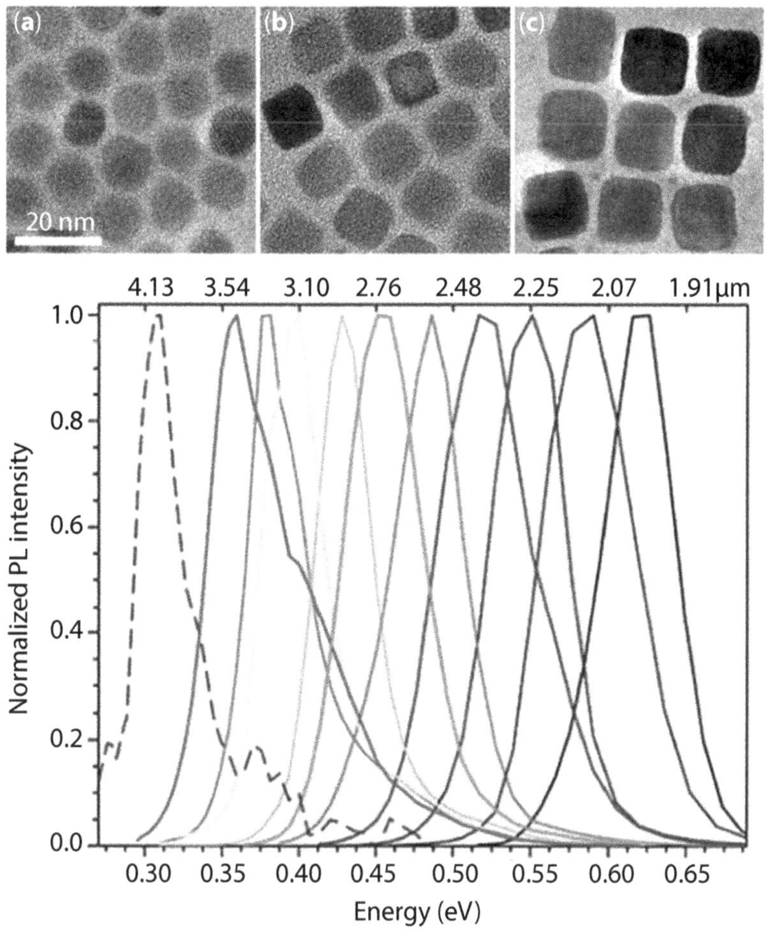

Figure 2.6 (Top) TEM images of size tunable PbSe quantum dots of (a) 11 nm, (b) 13 nm and (c) 16 nm. (Bottom) Normalized photoluminescence spectra of size tunable PbSe quantum dots. [20]. Reprinted with permission from [20]. Copyright 2004 American Chemical Society.

motion. The magnetic moment of an atom is given by the product of Bohr magneton, the g-factor and total angular momenta (J = L + S). For a free electron, being g = 2 and J = 0 + 1/2, the magnetic moment is one Bohr magneton, thus an element can show non-zero magnetic moment if it has non-zero spin. This is the case of elements with odd number of electrons, as some transition metals within d-shells partially filled, or rare earths within f-shells partially filled.

Roughly, materials can be classified according to their magnetic susceptibility, a dimensionless quantity defined as the ratio between the magnetization of the material in response to an external magnetic field H: $k = M/H$ where M is magnetization of material and H is the magnetic field. If k is positive the material is ferromagnetic, while if k is still positive but small (10^{-3} to 10^{-5}) the material is paramagnetic. When k is negative the material is diamagnetic. Note that compounds and alloys can be magnetic only if made by at least one magnetic element, with the exceptions of some alloys, like $ZrZn_2$ which can carry non-zero magnetic moment although made of diamagnetic elements (Zr and Zn).

For bulk materials, magnetism still arises from the electrons' spin. In this case, owing to the huge number of the overlapping atomic orbitals, band theory must be considered. In order to calculate whether the d orbitals are filled, the overlaps between s and d orbitals together with the exchange energy have to be considered. Indeed, exchange energy creates a spin imbalance in the band, since parallel and antiparallel spins interacts with different energy. Thus, the band splits into spin up and spin down bands with different amounts of electron [21].

Following Sorensen description, Nickel is employed as model for calculating the magnetic moment of matter. Nickel atoms have 8 electrons in the 3d orbital, and 2 electrons in the 4s. Without considering the exchange energy, the d band of Nickel in the bulk metal state is filled up to 9.4 electrons. Thus, it is a not completely filled band. By considering the band splitting, the 9.4 electrons of Nickel are distributed: 5 in spin up band (completely filled), and 4.4 in spin down band. Thus, an imbalance of 0.6 electrons creates a magnetic moment of 0.6 Bohr magnetons. The magnetic moments of adjacent elements in the periodic table, is easily quantified by adding or removing electrons from d band. For example, cobalt has 1.6 vacancy and iron 2.6. Moving right on the periodic table, copper has an excess of 0.4 electrons, which means that the d band is completely filled, and no magnetic moment is carried. By linearly applying this theory, it is possible to predict the magnetic moment of alloys with good accuracy.

At the nanoscale, however, magnetic properties of materials can completely change from the bulky state. For example, even diamagnetic bulk materials can carry a magnetic moment when at the size of NPs and the phenomenon of super-paramagnetism arises.

To understand the origin of size-dependent behavior of magnetism in nanomaterials, the domain wall theory of Weiss has to be considered [22]. A macroscopic ferromagnetic material, such as iron, has no magnetic moment in absence of an external field because it breaks into domains of a certain number of parallel spins and antiparallel spins to minimize the magnetic energy. This energy depends linearly to the volume extent of the spin domain, which is the physical volume through which the field extends. In theory, smaller and smaller domains can be considered to minimize the magnetic energy.

However, spin flipping requires energy in a ferromagnetic material which tends to align spins with parallel orientations. Thus, the creation of small domains with parallel spins jointly decreases the magnetic energy and produces an interface between oppositely oriented spins: a domain wall. The exchange of energy between two antiparallel magnetization directions is unfavorable in ferromagnetic materials. The result

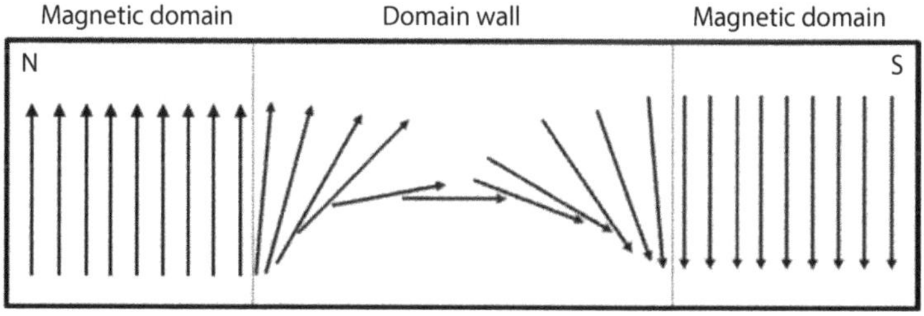

Figure 2.7 Scheme of domain wall creation between two opposite-spin magnetic domains.

is that many spins share the 180° flip in a domain wall of finite thickness. At the same time, in the domain wall, spins are not along the easy axis, defined as the direction of spontaneous magnetization, generating an energetic unfavorable magnetic anisotropy (Figure 2.7). The interplay between the exchange energy, that promotes the creation of thick domain walls, and magnetic anisotropy, that tends to minimize the domain thickness, results in the optimal magnetic domain thickness (typically of tens of nanometers).

At the nano-level, the size of nanoparticle is comparable to one spin domain. Hence, domain walls are not generated and single magnetic domain produced. Therefore, nanomaterials acquire magnetic properties that are not present at bulky state. One of the peculiar magnetic properties arising at the nanoscale in single domain NPs, is the phenomenon of superparamagnetism, which here is qualitatively described. Single magnetic domains can be considered such as unique giant spins with a bigger magnetic moment with respect to atoms. Indeed, each nanoparticle is composed by thousands of atoms. Supposing, for simplicity, that the magnetic anisotropy K is uniaxial, there are two possible orientations for spontaneous magnetization: at an angle of 0 or π with the easy axis. The two states are separated by an energy barrier KV, where V is the volume of the magnetic domain. The time needed for spin flip is called relaxation time. If the magnetization is collected at time steps larger than this time, a total zero magnetization is observed and the material is the superparamagnetic state. If the magnetization is collected before the relaxation, a blocked magnetization at its initial state is observed: this is called blocked state. Superparamagnetism can be experimentally observed by exploiting the relaxation time- and temperature-dependence. Magnetization measurements at a fixed time, by varying the temperature, are required to identify both the blocked and the superparamagnetic states. On the other hand, measuring the magnetization of NPs in response to an external magnetic

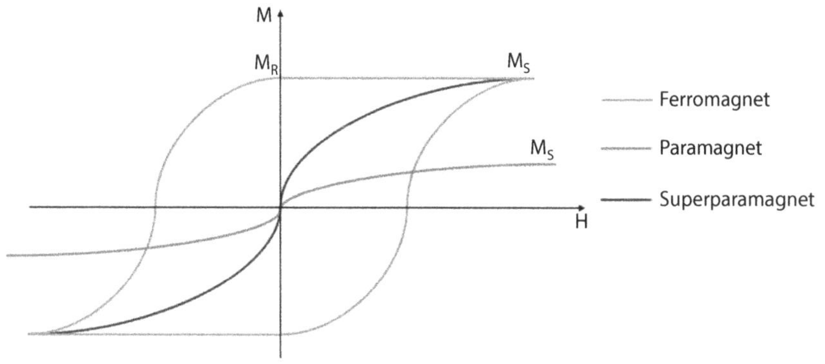

Figure 2.8 Langevin plot of magnetization (M) vs applied magnetic field (H) for ferromagnetic, paramagnetic, and superparamagnetic materials. M_S and M_R denote saturation magnetization and retentivity, respectively.

field at different temperatures is required in order to generate Langevin universal curves [23]. Superparamagnetic NPs show a steeper magnetization and a higher saturation magnetization with respect to paramagnetic ones, and have no hysteresis, as shown in Figure 2.8.

However, magnetism at the nanoscale is not only affected by the size of NPs (comparable to spin domains). Indeed, magnetic properties of NPs are also related to the increased surface/volume ratio, resulting in narrowing the d-bands. This behavior, such as for optical and thermodynamic features, is related to the atoms on the NPs surface that experience less coordination, which traduces in less overlap between d-orbitals and consequently increase in the density of states in d-band and magnetism.

Magnetism in NPs is also affected by ligands on their surface [24]. For example, electron donor/accepting ligands on paramagnetic NPs modify the population of the d-band suppressing or enhancing the magnetization (or creating surface magnetic anisotropy) by pumping or removing electrons from the particle. In this regard, an interesting example is related to the magnetic behavior of gold (diamagnetic in the

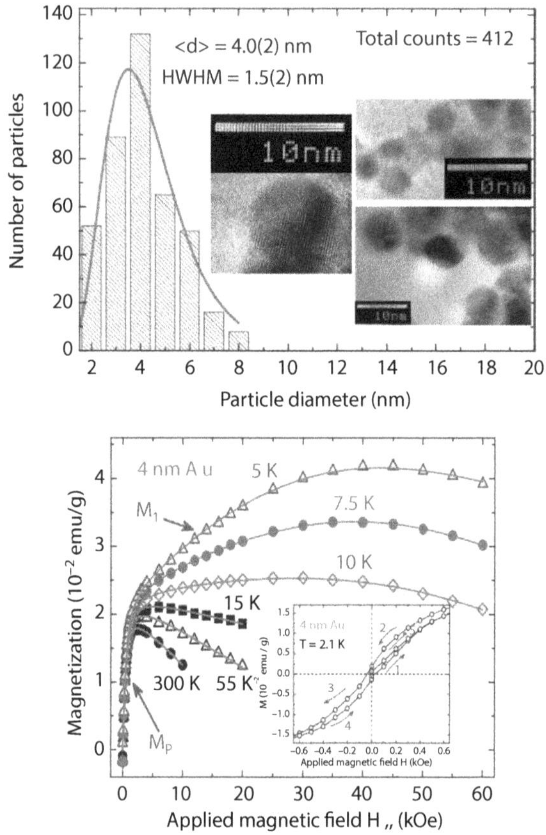

Figure 2.9 Magnetic behavior of bare gold NPs. Electron microscopy characterization of NPs (left) and magnetic response to applied magnetif field at different temperatures (right) [26]. Reprinted with permission from [25]. Copyright 2011 by the American Physical Society.

bulk) as ultrasmall NPs. Permanent magnetism is observed in polymer or thiol coated gold NPs [25]. This behaviour is associated to the 5d localized holes created by the charge transfer through the semi-covalent Au-S bond, which generate unoccupied state densities on Au surface, and then ferromagnetism.

It is interesting to notice that ~~also~~ bare ultrasmall Au NPs also show intinsic magnetic moment (Figure 2.9) [26]. These findings,

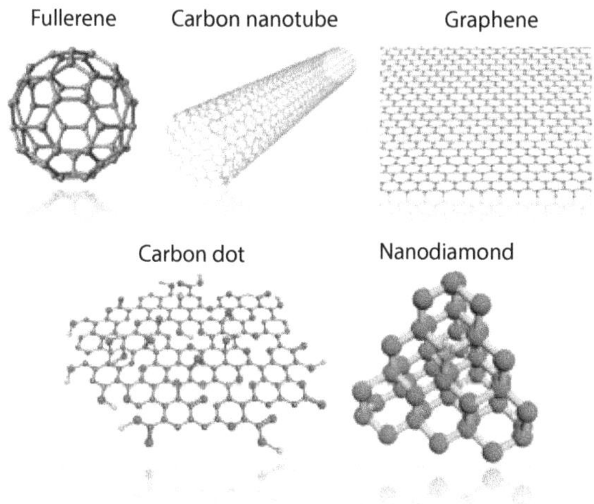

Figure 2.10 Schematic rappresentation of low-dimensional carbon materials [27]. "Reprinted with permission from [26]. Copyright 2015 American Chemical Society."

reported by Li *et al.* in 2011, are of particular interest since this behavior can't be attributed to ligand-mediated electron exchange, but exclusively to size reduction. Indeed,magnetic susceptibility measurements performed at many representative temperatures for various packing fractions of the nanoparticle assembly have showed that electron redistribution in the 5d bands were triggered by interparticle interactions which directly affected the magnetic moments of Au NPs.

Overall, size reduction to the nano-range results in the modification of a number of physical behaviours of the materials. Important properties such as thermodinamic, magnetic or optical ones become hardly predictable and several interesting phenomena arise. Getting insight on how nanomaterials behave has provided benefits in many aspects of daily life. In the following we will briefly discuss the most important achievement in the manipulation of the matter at the nanoscale, presenting an overview of the most popular nanomaterials, their synthesis routes and some important physiochemical properties.

2.2 Nanomaterials: An Overview

2.2.1 Organic Nanoparticles

Carbon

Carbon nanomaterials have attracted great interest in the last decades owing to their amazing physical properties that arise from quantum confinement, when the dimensionality lowers from bulk carbon materials such as diamond and graphite, to 2D, 1D and 0D materials (Figure 2.10).

C_{60} fullerene, a highly symmetrical carbon sphere made of sp2 carbon atoms, is the first carbon-based nanostructure that has received popular interest since its discovery in 1985 [28]. Like many other nanomaterials, it has been synthesized by top down approaches, (*e.g.* laser or heat induced evaporation of graphite), or bottom-up chemical synthesis from aromatic precursors. Fullerenes were proposed in the medical field as therapeutics and diagnostics when the water insoluble C_{60} molecules have been covalently functionalized with hydrophilic surface groups, increasing also their biocompatibility. Indeed, the hollow cavity of the C_{60} spheres is appealing for their loading with drugs or other moieties for diagnostics purposes. Furthermore, the unique photochemical features of C_{60}, among which the production of reactive oxygen species (ROS), increased the interest on these structures as oncologic therapeutics [29].

Sp2 carbon atoms at the nanoscale can also form tubular nano-objects (Carbon NanoTubes, CNT) made of either a single graphitic sheet, resulting in single-walled CNTs (SWCNTs), or multiple coaxial tubes, resulting in multiple-walled CNTs (MWCNTs).

SWCNTs physical properties depend on the direction in which the graphitic sheet is rolled-up, resulting either in semiconductor or metallic behaviors. In particular, semiconducting SWCNTs are of great interests in medicine for their ability of absorbing photons at bandgap energy and radiatively re-emit the absorbed energy as fluorescence in two NIR windows (650–950 nm and 1000–1350 nm) which are also known as first and second biological windows [30]. These ranges are of particular interest in medicine, because biological tissues are less prone to interact with photons at these energies, behaving as transparent [31].

Another important property of CNTs is their mechanical stiffness, which make them ideal candidates for tissue engineering or as scaffolds for tissue and nerve regeneration [32].

A much younger low dimensional carbon material is graphene, a 2D film of hexagonally arranged carbon atoms, whose discovery occurred in 2004 [33]. Graphene has been synthesized by a number of processes, including mechanical and chemical exfoliations, bottom-up epitaxial growth, and chemical synthesis. Graphene was the milestone for the revolution of electronics and photonics, owing to its high electrical conductivity [34]. It was also proposed as medical tool, being employed as biosensor with extremely high sensitivity [35, 36]. Furthermore, smaller forms of graphene, such as graphene oxide (GO) or reduced graphene oxide (rGO) has paved the way for graphene employment as drug delivery tool. Graphene derivatives (GO and rGO) have also shown interesting physical properties exploited for both therapy and diagnostics purposes (*i.e.* theranostics). These properties include tunable fluorescence emission, light absorption in the UV-NIR range, and peculiar ultrasounds absorption and dissipation [37].

Carbon Dots (or graphene quantum dots, CDs) are another class of carbon nanomaterials, that can be described as NPs whose chemical composition is carbon, oxygen, hydrogen and nitrogen with variable percentages. CDs have demonstrated a number of features similar to graphene oxide, including fluorescence from UV to NIR and up-conversion [38, 39]. Carbon dots can be, somehow, considered as the organic counterpart of semiconductor QDs. Carbon NanoDiamonds (CNDs), are the only carbonaceous nanomaterials showing a sp3 hybridization

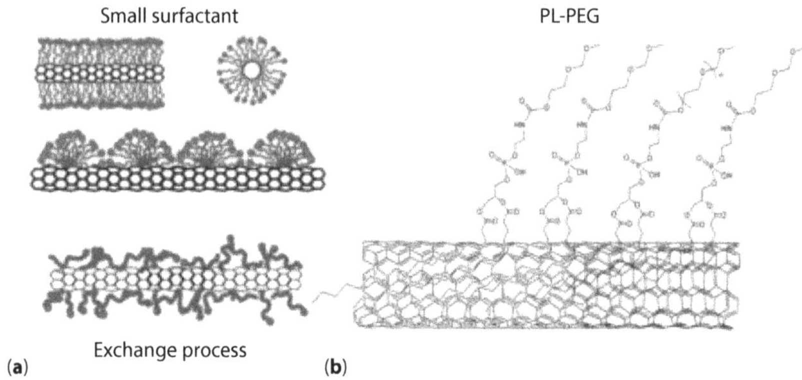

Figure 2.11 Surface functionalization of carbon nanomaterials by self-assembly of amphiphilic molecules (a) and by pi-stacking interactions (b). a) is reprinted with permission from [156]. Copyright 2015 American Chemical Society. b) is reprinted with permission from [27]. Copyright 2015 American Chemical Society.

of carbon atoms. CNDs size ranges from 2 to 10 nm. CNDs, such as CDs, are carbonaceous fluorescent NPs, but in this case, their fluorescence is peculiar and due to defects caused by nitrogen vacancies, which confers them tunable fluorescence in the visible range. These vacancies also provide dangling bonds which are exploited for chemical functionalization [40].

Carbon nanomaterials are often functionalized to make their surface more hydrophilic and biocompatible. Many strategies have been developed to covalently or non-covalently modify carbon surface, but for each kind of nanomaterial, a different strategy must be employed. Strategies employed for non-covalent surface functionalization include π–π stacking and hydrophobic interactions, which simply create micelles around the carbon nanomaterial (Figure 2.11). The main advantages of this kind of functionalization are the straightforward processes employed [41–43]. In particular, GOs and CNTs have been successfully non-covalently functionalized with electrically charged surfactants, as sodium cholate, CTAB, phospholipidis-PEG-NH2 (or –COOH), DNA, proteins, Triton-X 100, which allowed carbon nanomaterials to be dispersed in aqueous environment.

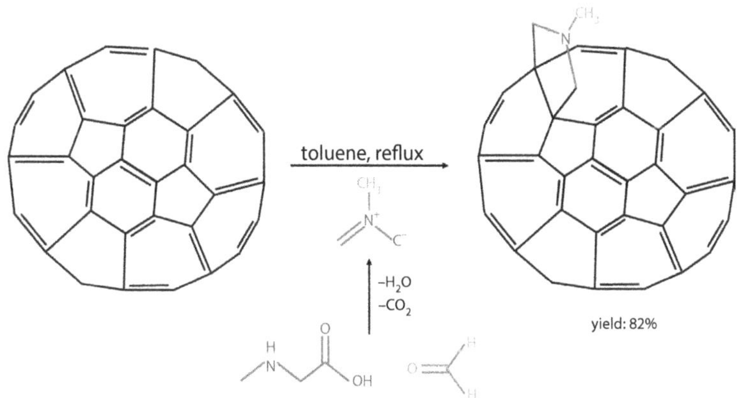

Figure 2.12 Scheme of Prato reaction for fullerene covalent functionalization.

Carbon nanomaterials can be also functionalized by covalent modifications [44, 45]. Many organic reactions have been developed for breaking the double bonds of sp2 carbon atoms and insert functional groups that confer the nanomaterials hydrophilicity and the possibility of further chemical functionalizations. As example, in Figure 2.12 is schematically shown the Prato cycloaddition reaction for the functionalization of fullerenes.

Carbonaceous nanomaterials can be treated by strong oxidizing agents, like H_2SO_4 or HNO_3, and in order to generate reactive carbonyls at the open ends which can be functionalized with amines or other functional groups. It is worth to note that all these reactions for covalent functionalization of carbon nanomaterials imply the modification of the pristine sp2 carbon surface, and this can have several implications in the physical properties of the material (*e.g.* electron conduction, lowered or impaired fluorescence quantum yield, or wavelength shift and enhancement of fluorescence).

Lipid Nanoparticles

Lipids are poorly water-soluble molecules composed by a polar end and a non-polar body which undergo supramolecular self-assembly in aqueous media. This self-assembly is driven by hydrophobicity which force amphiphilic molecules to expose the polar end of the molecule to water, confining the non-polar part into the core of the micelle. Vice versa, when amphiphilic molecules are injected in non-polar solvent, inverse micelles are obtained. In inverse micelles, the polar groups are in the core and the non-polar part of the lipid outside. The size of the micelles can be controlled by both the nature of the amphiphilic molecules and the environment conditions, among which lipid concentration, temperature or pH.

If two or more different amphiphilic molecules are injected together into a solvent, hollow spheres called vesicles are produced, whose shell is a bilayer (unilamellar vesicles) or more bilayers (multilamellar vesicles). A number of lipids can be employed to create vesicles. When phospholipids are used, the micelles are called liposomes, as proposed by Bangham in 1961 (Figure 2.13) [46]. Production of lipid vesicles can

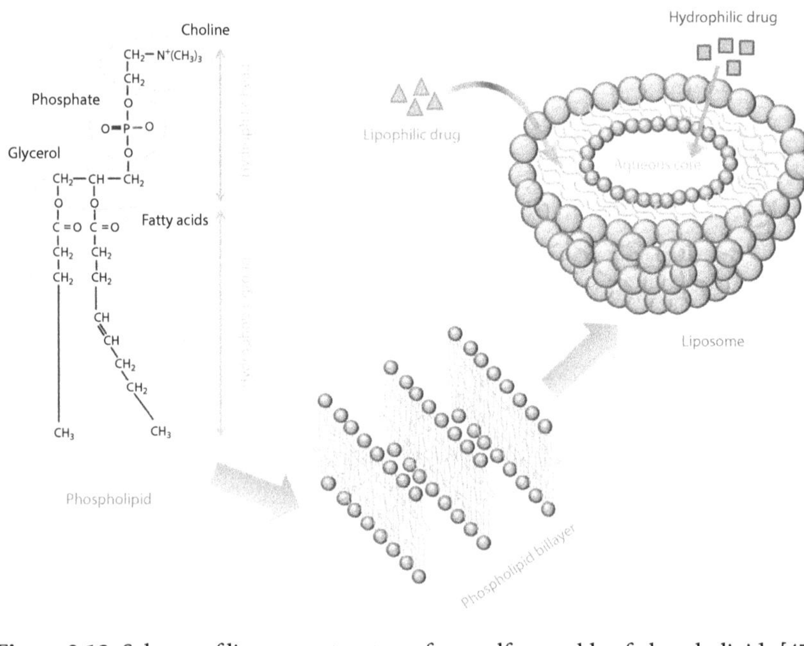

Figure 2.13 Scheme of liposome structures from self-assembly of phospholipids [47].

be achieved either through spontaneous self-assembly or by means of mechanically induced formation. The mechanical stress requires external energy to create the vesicles, and can be induced by sonication or extrusion techniques. Liposomes are today produced with a strong control over size (small, large and giant vesicles), number of layers (uni- or multi-lamellar) and size dispersion.

The original method for liposomes production proposed by Bangham was based on the hydration of a thin lipid film under agitation, which produced liposomes with a high level of polydispersity (both in size and number of lipid layers) [48]. Various techniques were adopted to reduce the dispersion and obtain smaller and more uniform vesicles. Some techniques involve the use of mechanical stress which degrades the lipid layers by promoting the formation of small uni-lamellar vesicles. Extrusion is the process in which multi-lamellar liposomes are forced through filters with defined pore sizes to obtain a liposome population with a mean diameter which is lower than filter pore. This process jointly yields to liposome size and lamellarity reduction due to the shear stress applied on liposome membrane by filter pore. Ultrasonication is another useful technique for producing liposomes with low lamellarity and size. In this case the shear force applied to lipid membrane is produced by cavitation. The main disadvantage of these techniques is the possible degradation of phospholipids [49, 50].

Also freeze-thawing belongs to the mechanical techniques category for the production of liposomes showing small size and lamellarity. Briefly, liposomes are snap-frozen in liquid nitrogen bath and gently thawed-up to the phase transition temperature of lipids. This strategy is also widely employed to exploit one of the most appealing properties of nanomaterials: the inclusion of moieties of interests, *e.g.* drugs, either in the central core or conjugated to the surface. In particular, freeze-thaw is an effective method for loading moieties in the liposomes through physical disruption of lamellar structure.

Ensuing ice crystals formation pores are generated in the lipid membrane and the drug that can freely diffuse to the area in which is less concentrated (*i.e.* liposome core). The diffusion mechanism is also thought to be coadiuvated by cryoconcentration, the phenomenon through which in a semi-frozen aqueous solution, the ice crystals are made of pure water, thus the solute molecules are expelled in the liquid phase which, in turn, results more concentrated [51].

A classical method to produce small vesicles without need for mechanical stress is the organic solvent injection in water. For this technique, lipids are dissolved in organic solvent (*e.g.* ethanol or ether) and they are injected into water in order to force the formation of vesicles. The main advantage of this technique is the production of highly concentrated water dispersion of liposomes. Indeed, the lipid solution is injected in hot water above the boiling temperature of the organic solvent, allowing its evaporation during the liposomes production. Usually, ether is preferred to ethanol as organic solvent because the latter is more difficult to be removed from water since it creates azeotrope.

A considerable advancement in the encapsulation efficiency has been made by the development of the reverse phase evaporation technique. Lipids are prepared in organic phase, and the solvent is then removed by rotary evaporation. This process affords the formation of a thin lipid film. Following, the film is dispersed in another organic solvent. Thus, a water solution of the molecule to be encapsulated is injected in the organic phase during sonication, leading to the formation of large unilamellar vesicles with high water/drug content. The organic solvent is then removed by rotary evaporation.

Another classical method to produce liposomes is by detergent dialysis. In this procedure, lipids are dissolved in aqueous media containing detergents. When the detergent is removed through dialysis, lipids forms large vesicles with high loading capability.

All these classical methods are straightforward, but demonstrate several drawbacks. In particular, the use of organic solvents can increase the toxicity of the vesicles, reducing their possible medical applications. To date, some methods to produce liposomes in large-scale and without employing harmful solvents have been proposed and detailed reviewed elsewhere [52–55].

Dendrimers

Dendrimers are a family of polymeric nanomaterials characterized by a symmetrical geometry. It is consistent with a central core from which branched polymers architectures develop in similarity to a tree (indeed the word dendrimer derives from the Greek word "Dendron", which means tree). Dendrimers are produced either with convergent or divergent approaches, as shown in Figure 2.14. The former consists of iterative coupling between monomers which have only one reactive site that can bind to their counterpart, and multiple protected sites that cannot react unless unprotected. In the convergent approach, the initial monomers will be in the end at the surface of the

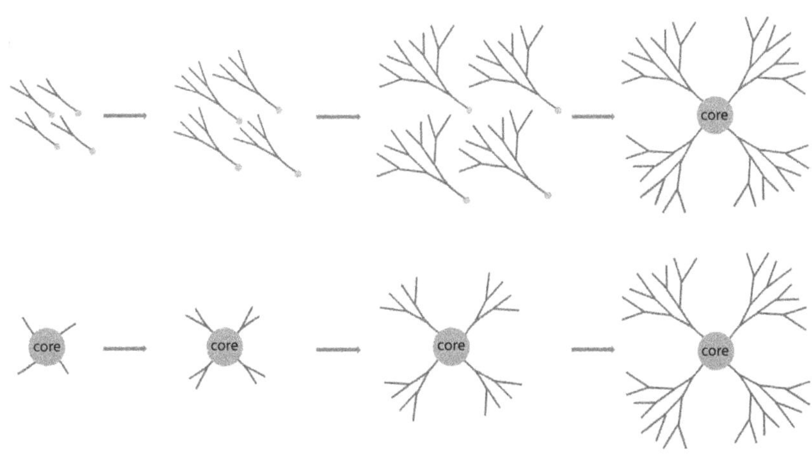

Figure 2.14 Convergent (a) and divergent (b) approaches for dendrimers synthesis [57].

dendrimer, and the growth reaction proceeds inwards, from the periphery towards a focal point and eventually ends on a center core. Each coupling step forms a "generation". Usually, the molecular weight of the dendrimer is doubled at each generation, since the number of coupling reactions is the same for each generation. Dendrimers produced with convergent approach are quite monodisperse, however there is a limitation in their maximum size owing to steric hindrance which impedes crowding of high generation dendrons around the core [56].

This size limitation does not occur in the divergent approach. In this procedure, the growth starts from a poly-functional polymer core with a certain number of active sites, to which monomers with only one reactive site and a number of protected ones are conjugated. At each generation, the diameter of the dendrimer increases, and the growth proceeds outwards. Usually, an excess of monomers is added to be sure that all the reactive sites have bound to their counterparts, thus purifications are required at each step.

The main disadvantage of divergent method is that at every step several precautions have to be taken in order to avoid side reactions or incomplete reactions, which can easily lead to defects (*e.g.* the branches of the final product have not all the same length). Furthermore, the purification steps to remove the unreacted monomers result time consuming if compared to the convergent approach. Regardless of the method employed, the final architecture of the dendrimers consists of: (i) a central core at which branches are attached, (ii) a branched structure which act as skeleton for the entire architecture, and can host drugs or other moieties and (iii) a multivalent surface, containing a huge number of active species which can act as grafting sites for drugs or targeting moieties. All these domains are tailored in response to the specific application needed, providing a huge variety of dendrimers with different size, surface charge, loading capability and active groups.

Among dendrimers, poly(amidoamine) (PAMAM), poly(propylenimine) (PPI), and poly(L-lysine) (PLL) dendrimers have been most widely studied, but virtually any other molecule could be organized in a dendrimer fashion, such as PEG and PEI polymers, or peptides. However, the majority of the monomers employed are cationic (bringing amines). This was the source of dendrimers high toxicity that it is due to strong ionic interaction with cell membrane. The acute toxicity is one of the biggest hurdles to be overcome for the widespread use of dendrimers for biomedical purposes. For this reason, many attempt of surface modification of cationic dendrimers by neutral or anionic molecules has been adopted, typically with hydroxyl or acetyl (neutral groups) and carboxyles (negative). On the other hand, modification with neutral or anionic moieties can impair the activities for which the dendrimers have been engineered for [58, 59].

Furthermore, toxicity is also related to the core employed for dendrimer growth. Indeed, many dendrimers are built on aromatic cores, which have hemolytic properties on rat blood cells, probably due to hydrophobic interactions with cell membrane [60].

Polymer NPs

Polysaccharides

Polysaccharides are polymers composed by sugars which have attracted enormous interests in nanotechnology mainly because of their availability in nature and abundance of reactive groups. Indeed, they can be found even in plants and animals and have a huge variety of molecular weights, which render them ideal low-cost candidates for the synthesis of multifunctional nanomaterials. Polysaccharides provides functional groups like amines and carboxyles, and can be further easily chemically modified to obtain specific non-toxic, biocompatible and biodegradable derivatives suitable for biomedical applications.

One of the strategies employed to produce polysaccharides NPs is the self-assembly of amphiphilic polysaccharides derivatives in aqueous environment. As an example, amphiphilic carbohydrates are easily obtained by chemical modification of the carbohydrate backbone with hydrophobic moiety. These derivatives are able to self-assembly as core-shell NPs in which the core is made by the hydrophobic-modified backbone and the shell is composed by the polar unmodified carbohydrates. Interestingly, they have shown appealing as platform for drug delivery of hydrophobic drugs, because these are confined in the central core of the nanoparticle [61].

Another strategy to produce polysaccharides NPs is the crosslinking (Figure 2.15). Crosslinking can take place either chemically or physically, by means of ionic interactions. Indeed, charged polysaccharides spontaneously crosslink to form NPs like aggregates in presence of oppositely charged cross-linkers, which can also be other polysaccharides. In physically induced aggregation, diagnostic or therapeutic agents can be trapped into the nanoparticle if dispersed in the same solution of polysaccharides. It is worth to notice that polysaccharides NPs can disassemble in response to environmental condition variations, like pH or ionic strength and this behavior could be efficiently exploited for endogenous triggered release [62]. Controlled aggregation can be also obtained by addition of chemical cross-linkers to carbohydrates, like glutaraldehyde, which interacts with polysaccharides functional groups. However, compared to physical crosslinking, chemical crosslinking has some drawbacks, among which the high toxicity of crosslinkers.

In the following, the most used polysaccharide NPs are briefly described, which are chitosan, dextran and hyaluronan, and the readers, if interested, are suggested to refer to detailed reviews [61, 62].

Chitosan is a cationic, linear polysaccharide composed of randomly distributed acetylated and deacetylated D-glucosamine

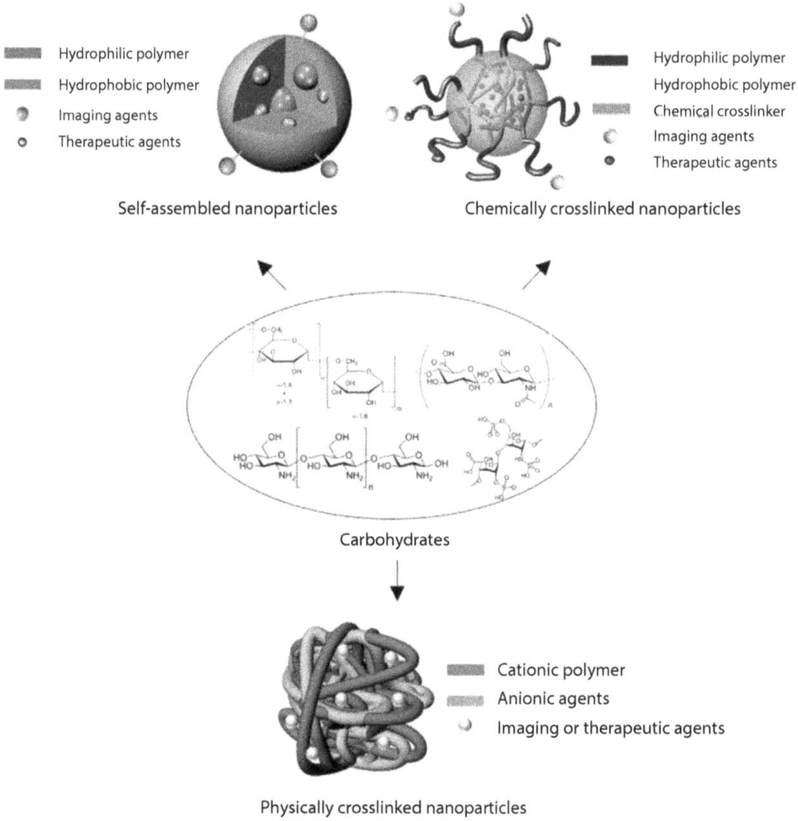

Figure 2.15 Scheme of strategies for synthesis of carbohydrates NPs either by self assembly of amphiphilic polymers (left) or by chemical (right) or physical (bottom) crosslinking [62]. Reprinted from [62] with permission from Elsevier.

units, linked through β-(1–4)-linkages. It is produced by deacetylation of chitin, a natural molecule present in the carapace of a number of animals. It is biocompatible and biodegradable. Moreover, the biodegradation products are nontoxic sugars which are reutilized by the body. As many other polysaccharides, chitosan NPs are produced by ionic or chemical crosslinkings [63]. Chitosan solubility in water is due to amino groups' protonation. Thus, it shows good solubility only at acidic pH. When amino groups of Chitosan NPs are coupled to drugs, which are often hydrophobic, their solubility in water is severely altered.

Thus, in order to produce NPs that are dispersible in aqueous media, chitosan NPs are often modified with hydrophilic moieties [64].

Dextran has acquired great interests for drug delivery applications, mainly as functional coating for drug carriers thanks to its capability to decrease opsonization effect in the bloodstream. For example, it was successfully employed as coating for metal NPs, in order to both improve their biocompatibility and as efficient targeting moiety towards early endosomes [65, 66]. The production of pure dextran NPs includes the employment of harmful chemicals, and the resulting NPs are poorly water-soluble. In order to increase dextran NPs solubility, dextran is usually conjugated with other polymers or polysaccharides, like chitosan. In order to improve the stability of dextran NPs in neutral and alkaline conditions, Iakobson *et al.* have recently reported a synthetic pathway for their production in water/ethanol mixture, resulting in NPs in the size range 150–450 nm (Figure 2.16) [67]. In this process, dextran is crosslinked with epichlorohydrin (ECH) and glycidyl methacrylate (GMA) in presence of ionic surfactant.

Hyaluronic acid (HA) is an anionic polysaccharide composed of repeating disaccharides of D-glucuronic acid and N-acetyl-D-glucosamine which is naturally found in human tissues, in particular in connective ones. HA has been extensively investigated in medicine for wound healing applications, as joint lubricant to ease osteoarthritis pains and also in oncology, since it bears the unique ability to bind cell-surface CD44 receptors which are overexpressed in a number of solid tumors [68–71]. Indeed, many drug-HA conjugates have been proposed for chemotherapy, including HA-Doxorubicin, HA-Cisplatin or HA-Paclitaxel [72–74]. Moreover, HA-proteins conjugates have been introduced, which showed enhanced proteins' blood circulation time [75].

In these conjugates, HA is mostly employed as targeting agent. The abundance of functional groups in HA is useful to be employed in the conjugation to amphiphilic or hydrophobic

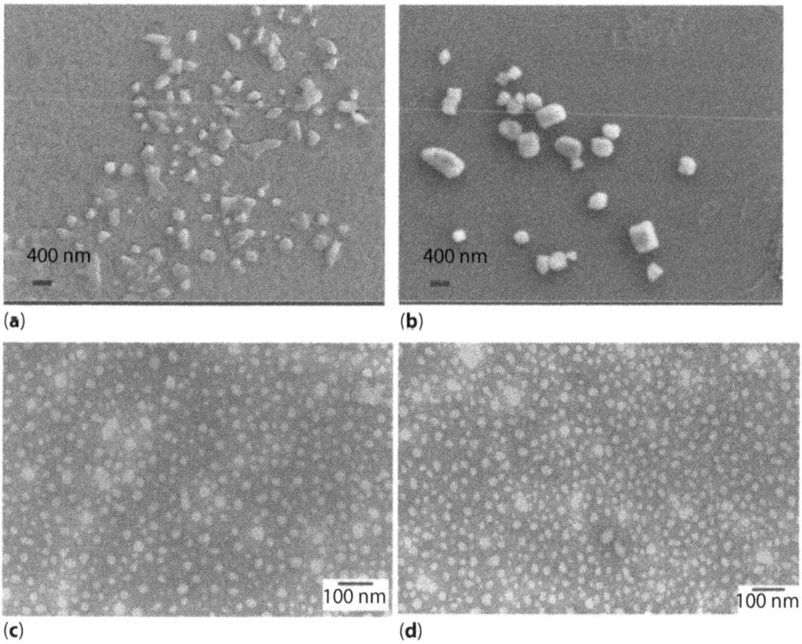

Figure 2.16 Electron microscopy images of dextran NPs obtained in aqueous solution (c) and in water/ethanol mixtures (a), (b) and (d) [67]. Reprinted from [67] with permission of John Wiley & Sons Inc.

derivatives, which allowed the production of self-assembled core/shell HA NPs in aqueous or organic media. Control over size and surface zeta potential of HA NPs is achievable by controlling the degree of substitution on the HA anchoring sites. Notably, compared to other polysaccharides, HA can reach high molecular weights and, upon crosslinking, it folds into an entangled network, in which the number of entanglements is highly dependent on the polymer concentration. This strictly-packed polymer network can mechanically entrap small molecules, drugs or even ultrasmall metal NPs, without the requirement of covalent linkage. This feature is very interesting since, by non-covalent encapsulation, the drugs can be entrapped in HA NPs without structural modifications, preserving all their therapeutic efficacy [76].

PLGA

Poly(lactic-co-glycolic acid) (PLGA) is a co-polymer consisting of poly(lactic acid) (PLA) and poly(glycolic acid) (PGA). It is one of the most widely investigated polymers in medicine owing to its biocompatibility. Indeed, it has been used for decades in surgery as material for sutures or prosthesis. The great success of PLGA is also attributed to its biodegradability. Upon hydrolysis, it depolymerizes in lactic acid and glycolic acid, two monomers which are naturally occurring in the organisms and that can be easily metabolized without producing significant systemic toxicity (Figure 2.17) [77].

In nanotechnology, PLGA has been extensively produced in form of NPs or nanofibers which were employed as scaffolds for tissue engineering [78]. PLGA is also an extremely versatile polymer since it can be finely tailored to the specific application. Indeed, by simply varying the percentage ratio of lactic and glycolic acid, biodegradation times can be tuned to grant, for example, sustained drug release over different timeframes. It is worth noticing that, by tuning the molecular weight of PLGA, its degradation times can be prolonged up to years [79]. Furthermore, it provides many anchoring groups which can be exploited for surface functionalization or drug loading.

Several strategies have been reported for the synthesis of PLGA NPs. One of the most commonly adopted is the emulsification – solvent evaporation technique, which consists in

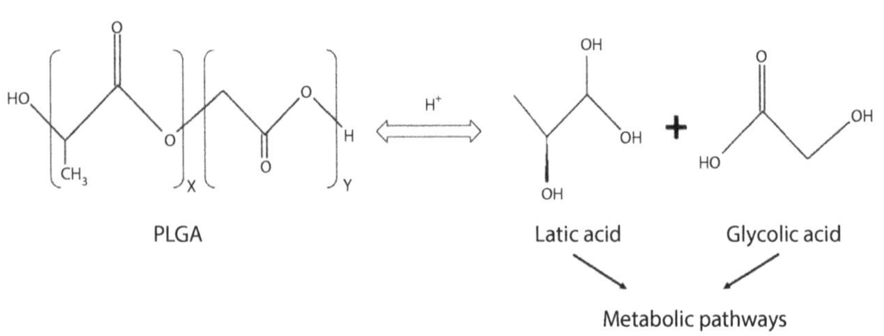

Figure 2.17 PLGA hydrolisis into lactic acid and glycolic acid.

creating oil in water (O/W) emulsion. O/W emulsion is created by vigorous stirring or ultrasonication of a mixture of PLGA dispersed in organic solvents such as chloroform or dichloromethane, together with water. Once the micelles are produced, the solvent is evaporated and the PLGA particles are collected through centrifugation. This technique is exploited for the encapsulation of hydrophobic moieties, such as drugs or dyes. A modified version of this technique, the double emulsion, allows the encapsulation of hydrophilic molecules, such as proteins or peptides. Briefly, the aqueous solution containing the drug is added to the organic phase containing PLGA and an emulsion is created. Then the emulsion is added to the aqueous solution containing the surfactant and the organic phase is evaporated, followed by the collection of loaded NPs [80].

Another technique for producing nanosized PLGA particles is by coacervation. When the aqueous solution containing the molecule to be loaded is injected in the organic solvent containing the polymer, an emulsion is created that is affected by parameters like temperature, pH, electrostatic repulsion etc. The addition of the molecule can decrease the polymer solubility by creating two phases: a polymer rich and a polymer depleted one. Gradual addition of organic medium to the polymer-drug-solvent phase while stirring, extracts the polymer solvent resulting in phase separation of polymer by forming a coacervate of polymer around the droplets containing the drug. To extract the microdroplets, the system is injected into a non-solvent. The final product can be extracted by means of solvent evaporation, for example with spray drying technique. In this process, the drug loaded NPs are put under a stream of hot air and the solvent is quickly removed [81].

Nanoprecipitation is another simple technique for producing NPs, which requires two liquid phases: the polymer solvent (usually organic or oil) and the non-solvent (water). When the solvent is added dropwise to the non-solvent phase under gentle stirring, a colloidal dispersion of nanocapsule

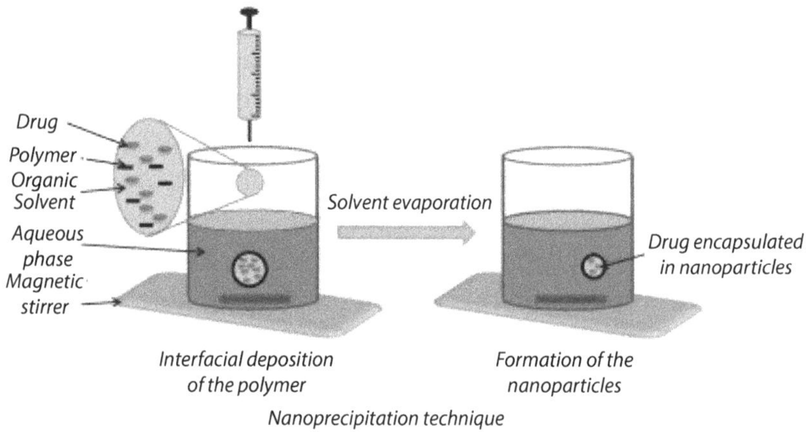

Figure 2.18 Schematic representation of nanoprecipitation technique [82]. Reprinted with permission from [82]. Copyright 2016 Springer Nature.

is obtained (Figure 2.18). Control over size and dispersion is obtained through optimization of polymer injection rate, stirring frequency, choice of the organic phase, drug and polymer amount and ratio between solvent and non-solvent phases. Supersaturation was described as the driving force of all these phenomena [82].

Polystyrene

Polystyrene latex (PS) is among the most popular plastic materials used for the production of biomedical devices or laboratory equipment, being inexpensive and biocompatible. It is an aromatic polymer which is naturally hydrophobic, but its surface can be modified in a number of ways to increase its hydrophilicity. PS NPs have been synthesized in a range of sizes and successfully employed as biosensors or in photonics [83]. Surface-modified PS NPs were used as probes for investigations upon protein corona formation on NPs in biological environment [84].

The most widely diffused synthetic protocol for PS NPs is the micro- or nano- emulsion polymerization, in which kinetically controlled polymerization of monomers is initiated by radicals and, once the NPs are created, they are stabilized by the addition of a surfactant (*e.g.* sodium dodecyl sulfate). This protocol is really simple and not time consuming since the monomers and the moieties to encapsulate are added to the reaction flask all at once before the radical polymerization is started [85, 86]. Some modifications to the protocol to synthesize PS NPs at nano-size range with improved monodispersion have been reported. In particular, Kim *et al.* have modified the synthesis of PS NPs by adding metal stearates to the styrene monomer solution. They showed that PS NPs with tunable size from 80 to 450 nm can be produced by varying the kind of metal stearate [87].

Unfortunately, only gut bacteria of mealworms are able to partially biodegrade PS latex polymer [88]. Furthermore, its degradation leads to styrene monomers which are harmful for human health and suspected carcinogenic. Consequently, there are no biomedical applications proposed for PS NPs.

2.2.2 Inorganic Nanoparticles

Metal NPs

Colloidal metal NPs are known since long time ago, when gold and silver NPs were used to decorate glasses. Starting from Faraday's work in 1857 and followed by the investigations by Ostwald, important progresses in understanding the basic mechanisms of colloidal NPs synthesis has been achieved. To date, researchers have a strong control over the physical or chemical synthesis of metal NPs. The fine tuning of their size and geometry is achieved, and a plethora of metal NPs has been introduced. In wet chemistry routes, metal NPs are often prepared in aqueous or non-aqueous solutions by reducing ionic metal from a precursor, typically a metal salt, with a reducing agent such as sodium borohydride, ascorbic acid, or trisodium citrate. This procedure is often carried out in presence of a coating agent, which stabilizes the colloid against aggregation and precipitation. Colloidal stability is achieved via electrostatic or steric stabilization by means of ionic or neutral capping agents.

Optimization of key parameters such as metal precursor concentration, temperature, pH, solvent, reducing agent, stirring frequency and even exposure to light, has to be taken into account to achieve precise control over size dispersion of the particles. This is a general rule for all kinds of metal NPs, in the following sections we will briefly describe synthetic routes and functionalization strategies for the most investigated metals, usually noble metals, and other metals which are recently emerging as promising nanomaterials for a number of applications.

Gold NPs

One of the most popular chemical routes for the synthesis of gold nanospheres was developed by Turkevich in the 1950s [89]. It is based on the reduction of chloroauric acid in aqueous environment by trisodium citrate, which acts both as reducing agent and ionic stabilizer. Based on LaMer mechanism, the production of NPs is a two-steps route: (i) the nucleation, where the precursor is rapidly reduced by creating a huge amount of "seeds" with narrow size distribution and (ii) the growth, or Ostwald ripening, where the size dispersion broadens because during the precursor concentration decrease, seeds directly contribute to the growth of larger NPs [90].

The size distribution of NPs can be controlled by modifying some synthesis condition. For example, by adding more precursor or performing the synthesis at low temperatures for delaying the ripening. The first option allows the nucleation to produce bigger and less size dispersed seeds. Today, by acting on temperature, gold precursor and pH, citrate capped gold nanospheres are finely tuned in the size range 3.6–200 nm (Figure 2.19) [91, 92]. The as produced Au nanospheres bear plasmon resonances covering the entire UV/visible portion of electromagnetic spectrum.

In order to synthesize anisotropic NPs, a symmetry-breaking condition has to be applied to the production method. This condition could be either physical (*e.g.* vigorous stirring) or chemical

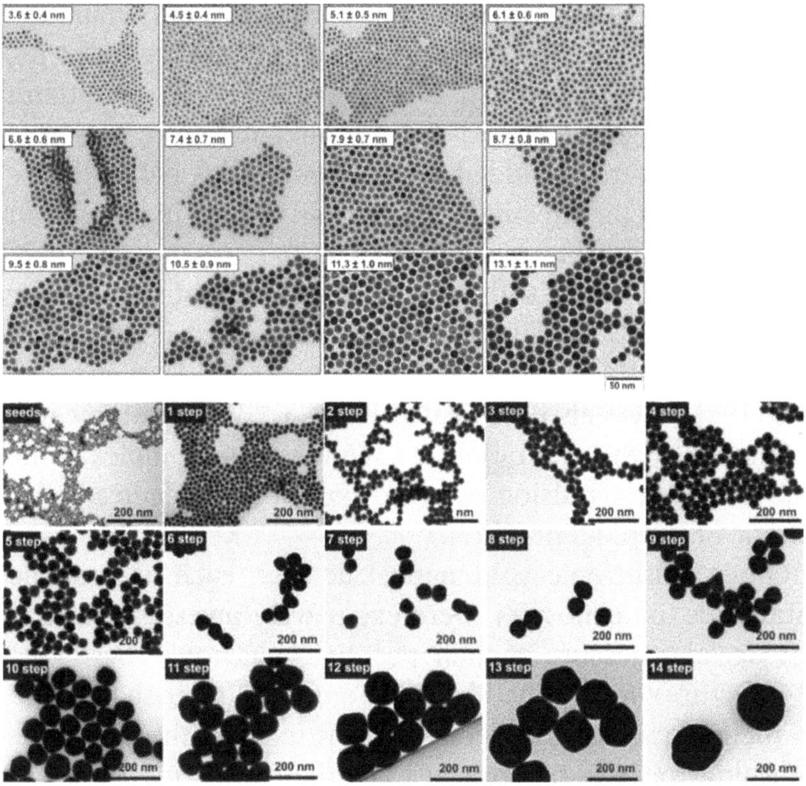

Figure 2.19 Transmission electron microscopy images of citrate-capped gold nanospheres with diameters ranging from 3.6 nm to 200 nm [91, 92]. Upper panel reprinted with permission friom [91]. Copyright 2016 American Chemical Society. Lower panel reprinted with permission from [92]. Copyright 2011 American Chemical Society.

(*e.g.* preferential adsorption of capping agent on certain crystallographic facets) [93]. Anisotropic gold NPs have been intensively investigated because they show LSPRs in the biological windows. In particular, gold nanorods with almost any size and aspect ratio in the nanometer range have been achieved by wet chemical synthesis after the introduction of the seeded growth protocol. Briefly, burst nucleation is performed by rapid injection of strong reducing agents to chloroauric acid. The seeds are subsequently added to the growth solution, where they act as nucleation centers. The most widely used capping agent for production of gold nanorods is cetyl trimethylammonium bromide (CTAB) which acts as a face-specific capping agent promoting uniaxial growth. It is demonstrated that any attempt to synthesize gold nanorods was doomed to failure if bromide counterions were not added to the reaction flask [94, 95].

Another factor affecting the synthesis of gold nanorods, and in general of anisotropic gold NPs, is the presence of $AgNO_3$ salt even if its role is still not completely understood. The longitudinal LSPR of gold nanorods is red-shifted if synthesized in presence of $AgNO_3$ because of the increase in their aspect ratio [96]. It was also speculated that CTAB elongation can be promoted by the generation of CTA+ AuBr4- complex, which can lower the repulsion between gold ions or decrease their kinetic of the reduction [97].

Other anisotropic gold nanostructures, such as branched multipods, or nanostars, were extensively investigated in the last decades because of their peculiar behaviors. These kinds of structures are highly desirable because of their sharp edges. In their proximity, the electric field is highly enhanced by the lightning rod effect. Moreover, multiple LSPR modes can be tuned by controlling the branch length. As to rods, the production of branched nanostructures is a seed-mediated synthesis, whereby the length and number of branches is finely tuned by adjusting the [seed]/[precursor] ratio. Branched nanostructures show multiple LSPRs: a weak band in the visible range (500–550 nm) which is attributed to the plasmon resonance of the spherical core, and an intense band in the NIR window (750–1000 nm) that is addressed to collective oscillation along the branches. Of particular interest are the five-branched gold nanostars. These nanostructures have plasmon resonances at wavelengths in the μm range, that can be reached by tuning the branch length (Figure 2.20) [98]. Their production was achieved by the same seeded growth synthesis protocol which leads to gold nanorods, but substituting CTAB with a non-ionic surfactant, Triton X-100. These structures showed two more LSPRs in

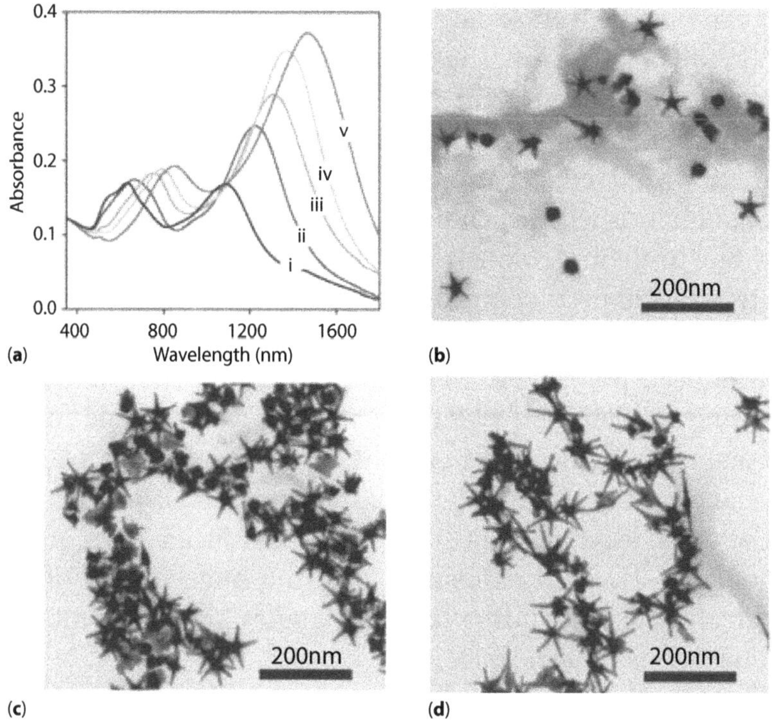

Figure 2.20 Extinction spectra (a) and TEM images (b-d) of gold nanostars with tunable size and branch length [98]. Reproduced from [97] with permission of The Royal Society of Chemistry.

addition to the core one at 500–550 nm, with one reaching the third biological window (1550–1870 nm) at 1600 nm. This portion of electromagnetic spectrum is of great biomedical interest as it allows for deeper light penetration in biological tissues and reduced phototoxicity. The presence of these LSPRs was attributed to the presence of co-linear branches allowing for longer longitudinal electrons oscillations.

Hollow gold nanoshells are another kind of interesting nanostructure for biomedical applications. The typical synthesis of gold nanoshells comprises a multistep procedure including a functionalization step on hard templates, the absorption of small seed NPs on it, and a seed growth step [99]. The template can be formed by silica, polymer or even metal nanospheres, and can be removed or not after the shell formation, depending on the optical properties required. The first two steps are of crucial importance for the final result since incomplete functionalization or poor seed coverage can lead to incomplete shell formation. Indeed, most of the published works present hollow gold nanoshells which partially resemble perfect shells, but very few of them demonstrate the optical properties matching the theoretical predictions of Mie theory.

Interestingly, hard template-free hollow gold nanoshells can be produced by APTES-in-water suspension [100]. By simply adjusting the [Au[3]$^+$] [APTES]/ ratio, it was possible to tune the diameter of the shells and the respective surface plasmon resonance in the range 657–957 nm (Figure 2.21).

The final kind of nanostructures introduced here are the nanoplates: 2D gold nanostructures in a huge variety of geometrical shapes, including circles, triangles, squares, pentagons and hexagons (Figure 2.22).

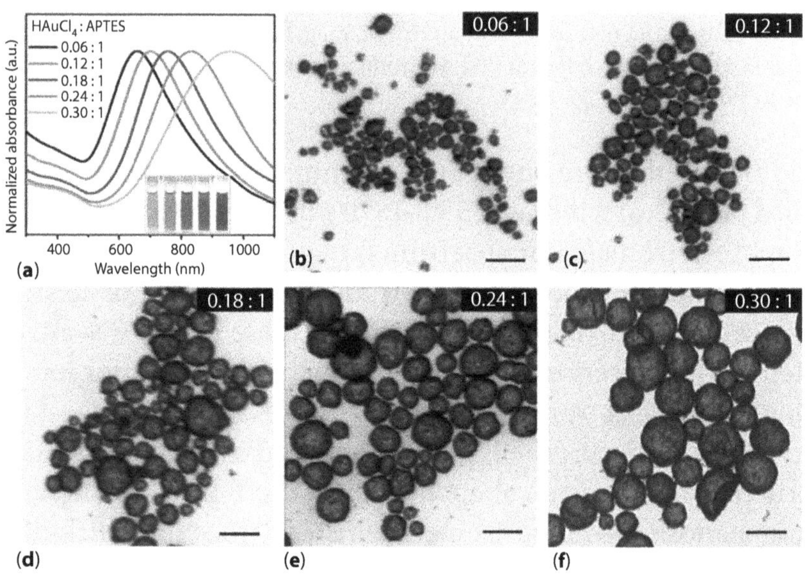

Figure 2.21 Template-free synthesis of hollow gold nanoshells with tunable diameter. Extinction spectra (a) and TEM images (b-f) [100]. Reproduced from [100] with permission of Elsevier.

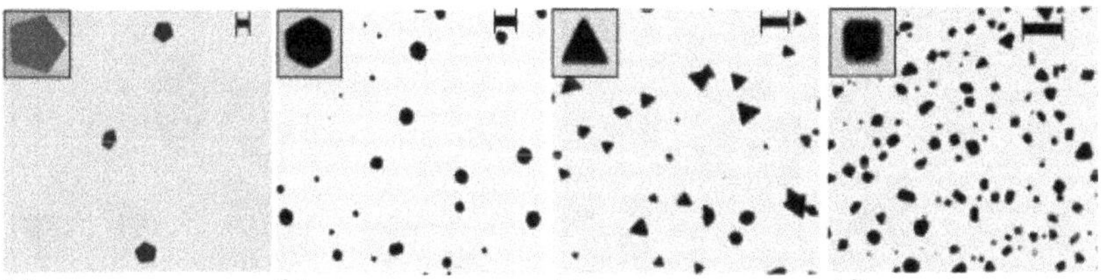

Figure 2.22 TEM images of polygonal gold nanoplates: pentagons (a), hexagons (b), triangles (c) and squares (d) produced by varying the synthetic conditions [101]. Reproduced from [101] with permission from The Royal Society of Chemistry.

Many synthetic strategies have been developed to synthesize 2D gold nanostructures, even if the seed mediated growth still remains the most popular due to its simple setup and relatively higher throughput. Notably, Chen and co-workers proposed a fast seedless growth approach for a high yield synthesis of triangular nanoplates by employing CTAC as surfactant and iodide ions (KI) as both etching agent and face-specific capping agent for promoting anisotropic growth [102]. Importantly, triangles edge length is finely tunable between 45 and 120 nm, as shown in Figure 2.23, with obvious implications in the plasmonic response.

An important behavior of Au NPs is related to their straightforward surface functionalization either through ionic or semi-covalent interactions. As-synthesized Au NPs usually show a surface charge related to the stabilizer used, *e.g.* citrate. Thus, oppositely charged molecule can be easily adsorbed to their surface by ionic interactions. Moreover, gold interacts strongly with thiols, generating semi-covalent Au-S bonds. This feature is employed in the ligand-exchange method, because the original surfactant on the Au NPs surface is replaced by other organic molecules containing a thiols (Figure 2.24) [103]. Moreover, thiolate molecules can be added *in situ* during the nanoparticle formation, in order to directly produce functionalized Au NPs avoiding a following decoration step.

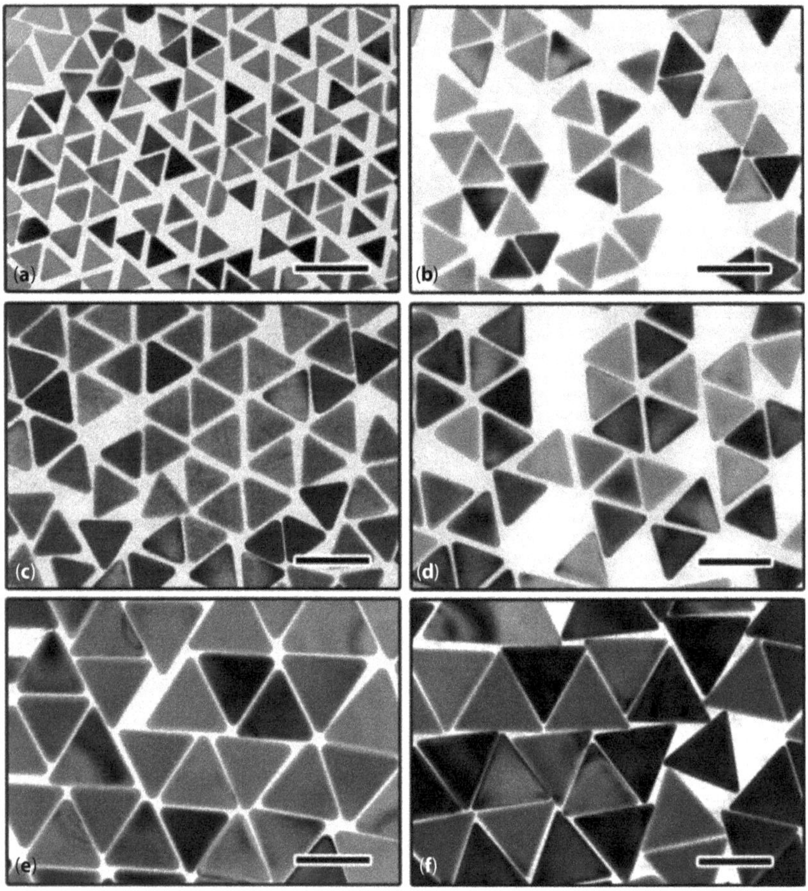

Figure 2.23 TEM images of edge length – tunable triangular gold nanoplates [102]. Reprinted with permission from [102]. Copyright 2014 American Chemical Society.

Ligand-exchange method has been used to decorate gold NPs with a wide range of ligands, including polymers (*e.g.* thiol-polyethylene glycol (PEG-SH)), dyes and drugs. Also engineered peptides composed by at least one cysteine have been employed to decorate AuNPs surface. The same approach can be also employed for proteins. Indeed, a number of BSA stabilized gold NPs were reported. On the other hand, proteins hardly retain their naive structure after interaction with gold surface. Thus, their employment is confined to stabilizer agents.

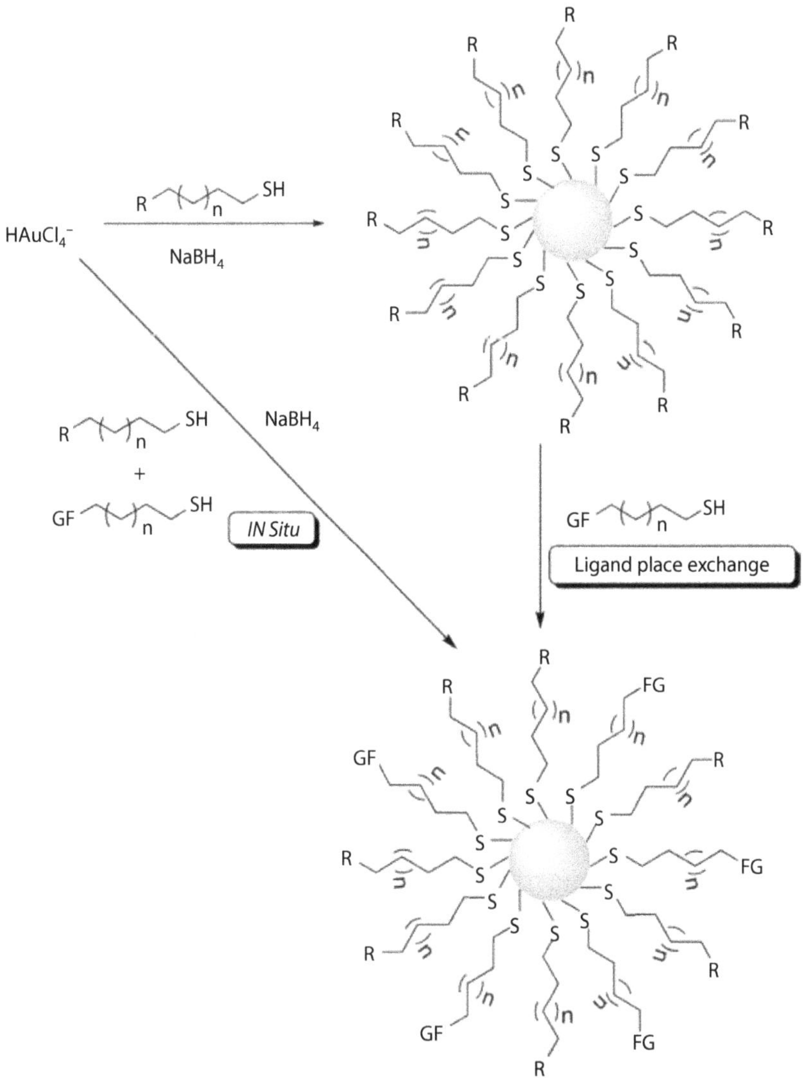

Figure 2.24 Scheme of ligand-exchange technique for gold NPs functionalization [103]. Reproduced from [103] with permission from The Royal Society of Chemistry.

The replacing coating has to provide to AuNPs at least the same stability of the mother surfactant, together with one or more functional groups. An efficient strategy for stabilizing gold NPs and conferring them functional moieties is the formation of self-assembled monolayers (SAMs) on their surface. SAMs are usually composed by polymers or peptides able to self-organize on the surface of AuNPs. These ligands are generally composite by an anchoring head (a thiol), a chain able to self-organize by non-covalent interactions, and final functional groups (amines and/or carboxylic acids). On this regard, gold NPs bearing both amines and carboxyl groups were successfully produced by replacing the original coating by engineered hexapeptides able to anchor to the gold surface by a cysteine and presenting to the environment the functional groups of a lysine [104, 105].

Silver

Together with gold, silver is the most investigated metal to produce NPs. As for gold NPs, small sized silver NPs are produced by a metal precursor and an excess of a strong reducing agent, such as sodium borohydride. Indeed, a burst reduction facilitates the creation of nuclei and impairing the ripening, resulting in the synthesis of monodispersed and uniform small sized silver NPs. On the other hand, to obtain larger-size NPs trisodium citrate is often preferred due to its mild reducing behavior [106–108].

Spherical silver NPs have been successfully synthesized by many groups, in particular, silver nanospheres in the range 5–100 nm were produced by dual treatment of silver nitrate with both slow and fast reducing agents, and the sphericity was controlled by pH tuning (Figure 2.25) [109]. Briefly, the first nucleation burst produced by sodium borohydride is followed by the growth of these nuclei by means of slow reduction of Ag cations by trisodium citrate, that also act as stabilizing agent.

Rainville *et al.* proposed a synthetic route for size tunable spherical silver NPs by the use of tannic acid and sodium citrate to reduce and stabilize silver atoms [110]. They achieved a controlled synthesis of silver cores ranging from 26–118 nm in diameter (Figure 2.26). Similarly, Bastus and co-workers obtained highly monodisperse sodium citrate-coated spherical silver NPs with controlled sizes ranging from 10 to 200 nm by

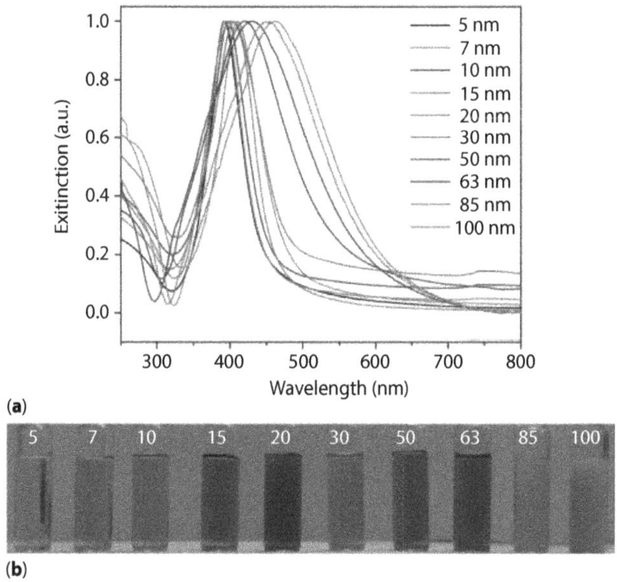

Figure 2.25 Extinction spectra (a) and colloidal solution photographs (b) of size-tunable silver nanospheres [109]. Reprinted with permission from [109].

following a kinetically controlled seeded-growth approach via the reduction of silver nitrate by the combination of sodium citrate and tannic acid [111]. In this seed-mediated growth, the homogeneous growth of Ag seeds is kinetically controlled by adjusting reaction parameters: concentrations of reducing agents, temperature, silver precursor to seed ratio, and pH.

Investigations on anisotropic growth of silver NPs led to the production of silver nanostructures of various shapes, including prisms, rods, shells, branched nanostructures and 2D plates. As for gold, when the structural symmetry is somehow broken, silver NPs suffer from drastic changes in their physical and even biological properties.

The majority of the synthetic routes for the production of anisotropic silver NPs are based on a seed-mediated growth in presence of face-specific strong surfactants which promote the anisotropic growth. However, synthesis of branched silver NPs (*i.e.* nanostars) has been achieved by reducing a silver salt with hydroxylamine and citrate, which operated also as soft capping agent [112].

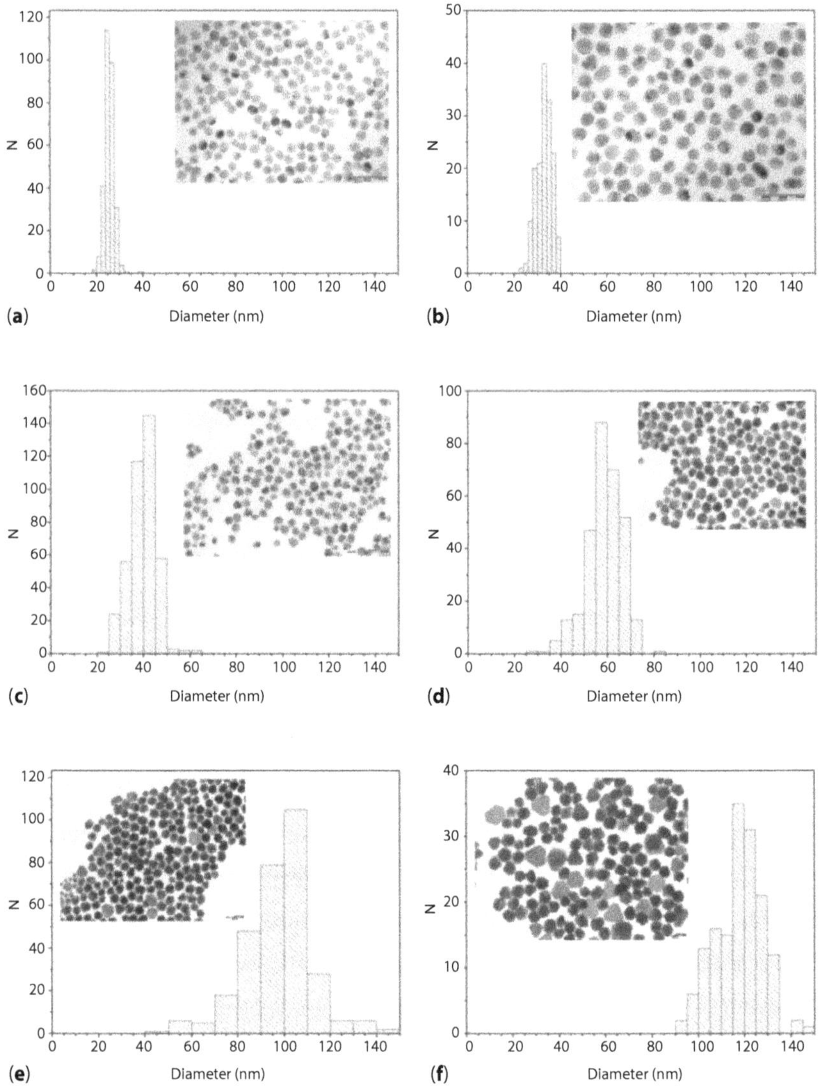

Figure 2.26 Size dispersion hystograms and TEM images (insets of size-tunable silver NPs of 26 nm (a), 33 nm (b), 40 nm (c) 59 nm (d), 96 nm (e) and 118 nm (f). [110].

Systematic investigations on the role of the reactives in the synthesis of silver nanoprisms, resulted in the production of nanoplates with finely tuned plasmon resonances covering the whole range UV/NIR (Figure 2.27) [113].

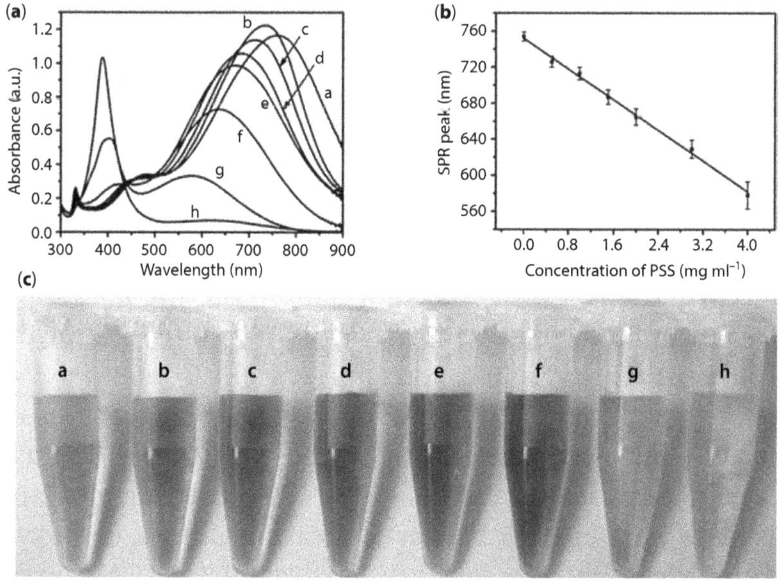

Figure 2.27 (a) Absorbance spectra of silver nanoplates synthesized with different concentrations of poly(sodium 4-styrene sulfonate) (PSS). (b) Absorbance maxima vs PSS concentration and (c) photograph of silver nanoplates colloidal solutions [113]. Reprinted from [113] with permission of Elsevier.

Many groups have achieved the production of non-spherical silver NPs by employing light-induced ablation, oxidation or coalescence. Lee and co-workers reported that in the photo-induced synthesis of silver nanoprisms, both the sizes of the original seed NPs as well as the overall photon flux are critical reaction parameters to determine the quality of nanoprisms [114]. Pietrobon *et al.* reported the synthesis of silver nanorods with pentagonal facets and tunable size by anisotropically reducing silver salts on decahedral silver seeds produced by exposing silver NPs to blue light for several hours [115].

A seedless synthetic approach for the production of silver nanorods of 20 nm in diameter and tunable length up to 100 nm was reported by El-Sayed [116]. In this approach, silver salts are reduced with ethylene glycol in presence of PVP as capping agent. The LSPR bands are centered at 400 nm for the transverse oscillation mode and cover the range 545–900 nm for the longitudinal modes, according to their aspect ratio.

Recently, great attention has been given to the synthesis of silver nanoshells composite on SiO_2 hard templates. The shell growth is reached either by employing the presence of ultrasmall silver NPs attached to the silica surface, or by a one-step direct reduction of silver precursors on thiol-functionalized silica surface in presence of octylamine [117]. Interestingly, the shell thickness, and thus the optical response of nanoshells, can be tuned in the seedless approach by simply varying the ratio of silver precursor to silica template, avoiding multistep growth.

The most widely employed capping agent for silver NPs is citrate which, as already mentioned for gold NPs, act also as reductant. Polymers like PEG, PVP and PVA were widely used for electrosteric stabilization of silver NPs. Moreover, inorganic, organic or even biological moieties bearing amines, carboxyles and thiols can be used for coating silver surfaces. Ag surface has also affinity to aromatic moieties like phenols, which were successfully employed to coat silver nanowires through covalent Ag-C bonds [118].

Platinum

Platinum is another well-investigated metal for the production of nanomaterials. As for gold and silver, many methods were adopted for the synthesis of Pt NPs, but, being an easy and almost inexpensive route, the chemical pathway is one of the most extensively investigated. The most common precursor used in platinum NPs synthesis is H_2PtCl_6 [119]. As usual, after the salt has been dissolved in water or organic solvents, a reducing agent is employed for the creation of Pt NPs.

Synthetic pathways for producing spherical Pt NPs ranging from ultrasmall NPs (1–5 nm) to monodisperse spherical NPs of 10–100 nm and the related optical properties have been reported (Figure 2.28) [120].

The introduction of foreign ions during wet-chemistry synthesis of Pt NPs is the major approach to control their morphology (some examples of anisotropic Pt NPs are shown in

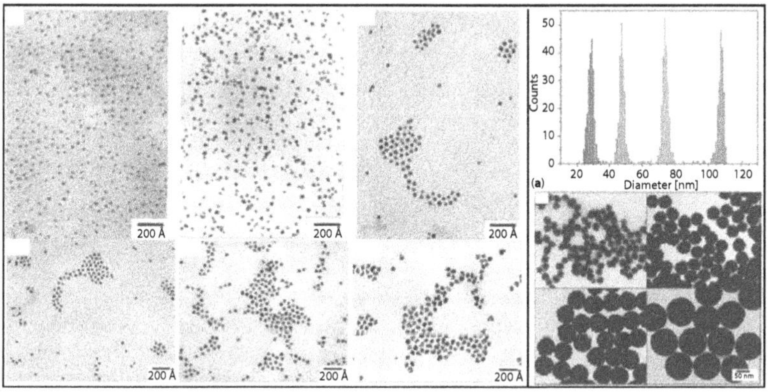

Figure 2.28 TEM images and size dispersion (top, right) of nearly-monodisperse platinum nanospheres [120]. (Left panel) Reprinted with permission from [170]. Copyright 1999 American Chemical Society. (Right panel) Reprinted with permission from [120]. Copyright 2008 American Chemical Society.

Figure 2.29). For example, silver ions preferentially adsorb on Pt facets leading to formation of truncated tetrahedra and cuboctahedra [121, 122]. Silver ions were also added to the Pt precursor solution, for triggering the synthesis of Pt multipods [123]. Other ions, such as Fe^{3+}, have been shown to promote the growth of single crystal Pt nanowires in presence of PVP and oxygen, however, the exact mechanisms at the basis of this behavior is not yet clearly understood. It is only speculated that selective adsorption of the foreign ions on crystal facets changes the rate of growth promoting shape anisotropy [124].

Compared to gold and silver, Pt NPs do not show sharp plasmonic responses in the visible or NIR range, but exhibit broad extinction bands in the UV part of the spectrum. Shifting the plasmonic response on visible wavelengths without increasing too much the size of Pt NPs and thus compromising their usefulness, is a major concern for this kind of nanostructures.

Other Metals

Wet-chemistry has been also successfully exploited for the production of NPs of other metals. The general principle is always

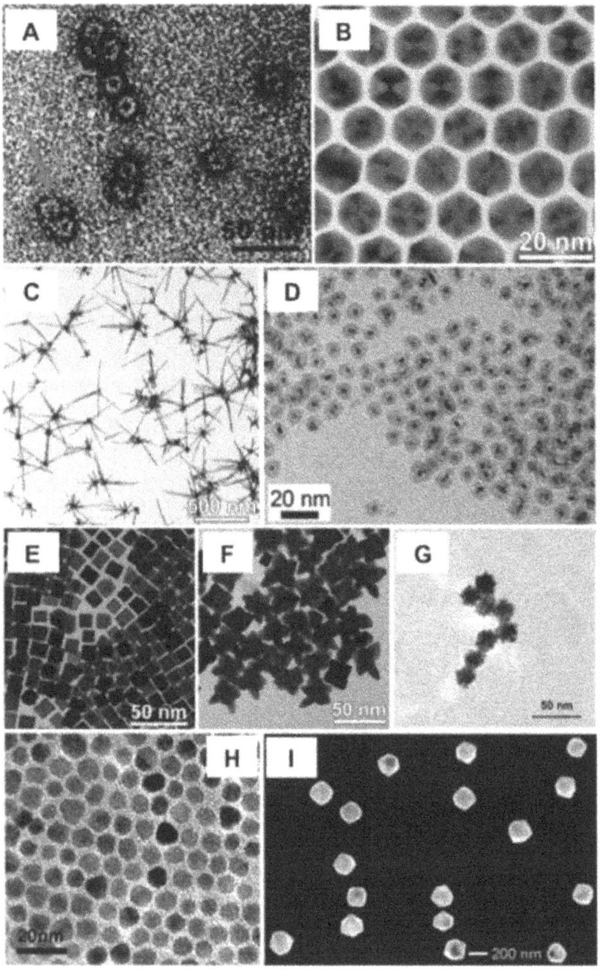

Figure 2.29 (a) Reproduced with permission from [157]. Copyright 2010 American Chemical Society. (b,c,e,f) Reproduced with permission from [158]. Copyright 2013 American Chemical Society. (d) Reproduced with permission from [159]. Copyright 2008 American Chemical Society. (g) Reproduced from [160] with permission of The Royal Society of Chemistry. (h) Reproduced with permission from [161]. Copyright 2005 American Chemical Society. (i) Reproduced from [162] with permission of John Wiley & Sons Inc.

the reduction of metal salts from ionic to metallic state, in presence of stabilizing capping agents.

Being an earth-abundant and almost inexpensive metal, copper has attracted great interests in many fields of science.

However, the synthesis of Cu NPs is challenging because the copper instability due to its propensity to oxidation, which makes it difficult to produce NPs under atmospheric conditions. Many efforts to increase the stability of Cu NPs avoiding the employment of argon or nitrogen atmosphere have tested, resulting in the introduction of complex Cu core/shell nanostructures resistant against oxidation.

Spherical Cu NPs shown a plasmon resonance is in the range of visible light, reaching a maximum of ~580 nm [126]. However, optical response of Cu NPs strongly depends on the presence of a shell composed by an oxide layer. Dang *et al.* reported a systematic study on this feature in a range of pH from 8 to 14, correlating the LSPR shifts to the decrease in size of the NPs or to the appearance of oxidized particles [127].

Cobalt NPs have been produced by reducing cobalt chloride or cobalt acetate in presence of strong capping agents and under nitrogen or argon atmosphere to prevent oxidation. In particular, ultrasmall Co NPs with low level of oxidation were successfully produced by reduction of cobalt chloride in DMSO as both solvent and capping agent [128].

Compared to noble metal NPs, Co NPs are non-plasmonic but possess a large magnetic moment, making them interesting materials for diagnostic purpose [129, 130]. Many groups have investigated the magnetic anisotropy of Co NPs, reporting size effects and also controlling the anisotropy level by finely tuning the oxidization state by exposing the Co NPs to atmospheric oxygen to grow an oxide shell around them [131].

Although LSPR is theoretically possible in any metal, alloy or semiconductor with a large negative real dielectric constant and small imaginary dielectric constant, only metal NPs with a sharp resonance in the visible range are of interest for medical applications.

In this regard Aluminum NPs are less investigated compared to noble metals like Ag and Au, mainly because: i) their tendency to oxidize, such as copper and cobalt, and ii) their optical properties (Al NPs of 40 nm have a plasmon resonance band centered in the UV region) which renders them not so appealing for medical purposes.

However, the LSPR shift in Al NPs due to their increase in size is considerably higher than in other metals, indeed it was calculated that the SPR of Al NPs will shift from 200 nm for 20 nm Al nanospheres, to the visible range for spheres of 140 nm. In particular, it was calculated that for anisotropic Al NPs (*e.g.* nanorods) the appearance of a sharp plasmon band at 495 nm would take place for the longitudinal oscillation mode [132].

Other plasmonic metal NPs which are receiving increasing attention are palladium, nickel and rhodium NPs. Pd NPs smaller than 40 nm in diameter do not show any plasmon resonance above 200 nm, while the ones with diameter over 50 nm show a single LSPR peak in the UV region. Pd NPs larger than 90 nm in diameter exhibit multiple resonances in the entire range UV-NIR, up to 1200 nm [133]. Planar tripods of 8 nm Rh NPs, were synthesized by a modified polyol reduction method and presented a calculated plasmonic response in the UV around 330 nm [134]. A broad plasmon resonance in the UV region was also predicted for Ni NPs, around 450 nm, but the increasing interest in these NPs relies in their magnetic behavior useful for magneto-optical devices, rather than in their plasmonic response [135].

Iron Oxide NPs

When metals undergo oxidation, they can form a huge variety of interesting compounds which, when tailored to nanoscale, can show interesting physical and chemical properties. Recently, many efforts have been devoted to fine tailoring metal oxide NPs, including the most investigated iron oxides, but also TiO_2, CeO, In_2O_3, ZrO, and Al_2O_3. Most of the synthetic routes are based on wet chemistry which are mainly performed in oxygen-containing organic solvents due to the high reactivity of oxides towards water [136].

Some of the organic solvents employed for the syntheses of metal oxides NPs are acetone, alcohols, toluene, benzylamine, which are often metal-specific. On the other hand, benzyl alcohol is an almost ubiquitous solvent which has been reported for the synthesis of more than 35 different metal oxides NPs [137].

Despite the plethora of synthetic pathways, the basic principle of metal oxide NPs synthesis is the condensation reaction, *i.e.* the formation of metal oxides monomers (metal-oxygen bond), where the oxygen is supplied by the solvent [138]. After the production of metal oxides monomers through condensation (examples of condensation reactions are reported in Figure 2.30), they undergo usual nucleation and growth processes common to all protocols for producing NPs.

Iron oxide NPs (IONPs) are, by far, the most extensively investigated metal oxides NPs. Iron and oxygen chemically react to produce sundry iron oxides such as magnetite (Fe_3O_4), maghemite (γ-Fe_2O_3), and hematite (α-Fe_2O_3). All of these compounds exhibit either ferromagnetism or ferrimagnetism at room temperature, and many IONPs showed super paramagnetic behavior (SPIONs), attracting great interests in medicine, mostly as contrast media for magnetic resonance techniques [139].

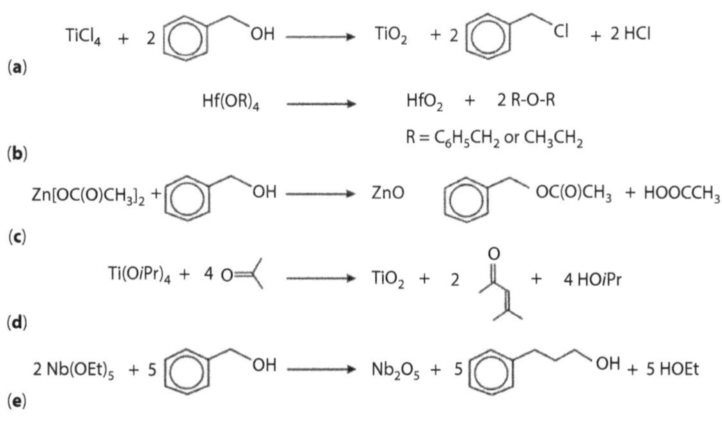

Figure 2.30 Examples of condensation steps to synthesize metal oxide NPs [138]. Reproduced from [137] with permission of Elsevier.

As already stated, direct synthesis of IONPs in aqueous media is challenging. Thus, the majority of reported syntheses were performed in organic solvents, and IONPs were subsequently modified to make them water soluble.

Monodisperse spherical maghemite NPs in the size range from 6 to 13 nm was reported by Hyeon, using iron chloride as precursor and oleate in organic solvent and by tuning the size of the nanospheres by optimizing the reaction temperature (Figure 2.31) [140].

High control over size and morphology of IONPs is a key-requisite, since size affects dramatically the magnetic properties of these nanomaterials due to size-dependent spin exchange effect. Moreover, controlling the shape of magnetic NPs can induce magnetic anisotropy that substantially affects proton spin relaxation times. On this regard, Zhou *et al.* have recently reported the synthesis of IONPs with various shapes, among which cubes, plates, tetrahedrons and branched nanostructures, synthesized by thermal decomposition of iron oleate in the presence of sodium oleate (Figure 2.32) [141]. These nanostructures were investigated as MRI contrast agents.

Stabilizing iron oxide NPs is crucial to avoid aggregation and precipitation of the colloids, due to their intrinsic magnetic behavior.

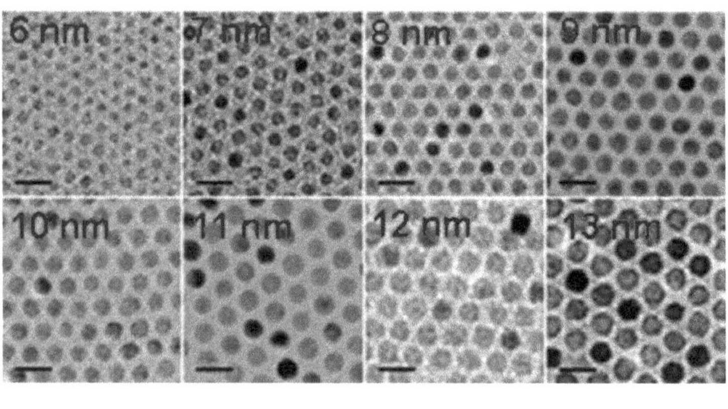

Figure 2.31 TEM images of monodisperse maghemite nanospheres with diameter ranging from 6 to 13 nm [140]. Reproduced with permission from [140]. Copyright 2001 American Chemical Society.

Electrostatic and steric stabilization has been widely employed for IONPs, by exploiting the affinity of iron oxide towards carboxyl groups, phosphates and sulfates. Coating with polar moieties, polymers and even PAMAM dendrimers provided at the same time biocompatibility and water solubility to IONPs [142].

Noble metals have been proposed as stabilizers for IONPs in order to develop smart nanomaterials. Indeed, engineered core/shell multimodal platforms for medical purposes can be developed by the growth of a noble metal shell on IONPs [143, 144].

Silica NPs

Silica, or silicon dioxide (SiO_2), is a class of materials composed by silicon and oxygen: the most abundant mineral on earth surface. It has been widely employed as constituent of glasses or in microelectronics. Nanosized silica is biocompatible, optically transparent, chemically inert and has an exceptional thermal stability. Most of the reported water-soluble silica NPs have been successfully synthesized in wet chemistry by following two main pathways: the Stöber sol-gel approach, and the reverse water/oil (w/o) microemulsion. Stöber process[145], proposed in 1968, involves the hydrolyzation of tetra alkyl silicates in a water/alcohol solution, in which ammonia was employed as catalyst. This process leaded to highly monodispersed silica NPs in the nanometer range, tunable up to microns by adjusting the reaction parameters (Figure 2.33).

Briefly, tetraethyl orthosilicate (TEOS) is hydrolyzed by water producing silanols groups which undergo polymerization by condensating with other silanols or with ethoxy groups creating siloxanes, according to the reactions:

$$Si\left(OC_2H_5\right)_4 + H_2O \xrightarrow{hydrolysis} Si\left(OC_2H_5\right)_3 OH + C_2H_5OH$$

$$\equiv Si - O - H + H - O - Si \equiv \xrightarrow{water\ condensation} \equiv Si - O - Si \equiv H_2O$$

$$\equiv Si - OC_2H_5 + H - O - Si \equiv \xrightarrow[\quad]{\substack{alcohol\\ condensation}} \equiv Si - O - Si \equiv + C_2H_5OH$$

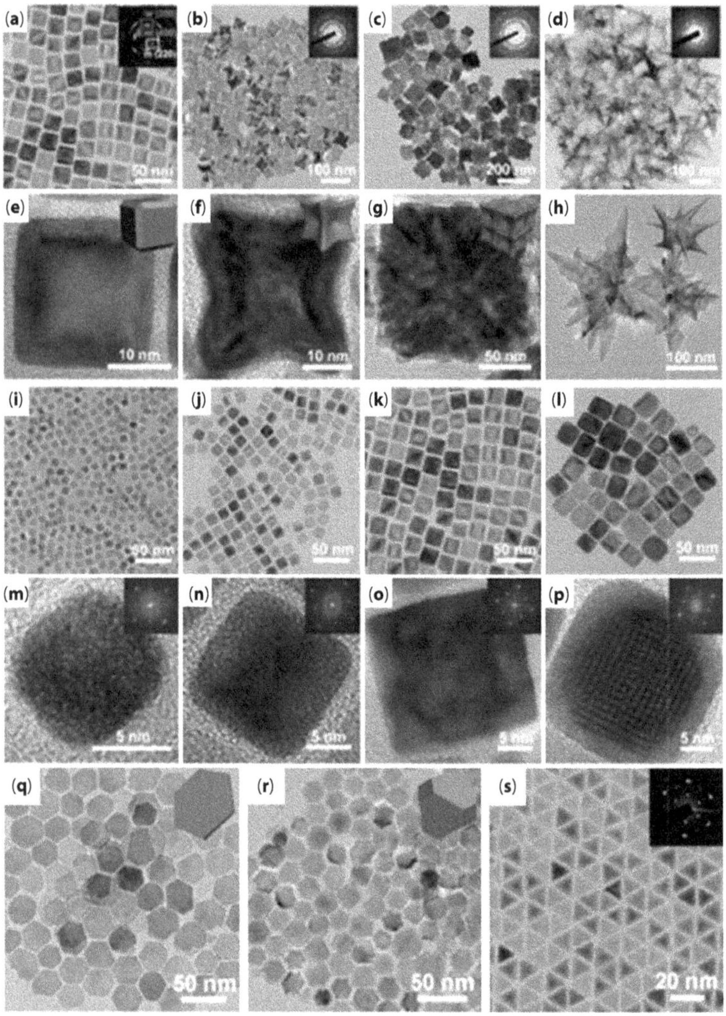

Figure 2.32 TEM images and 3D structure (insets) of anisotropic iron oxide NPs [141]. Reproduced with permission from [141]. Copyright 2015 American Chemical Society.

Hydrolysis of TEOS produces orthosilicic acid, whose polymerization occurs when its concentration exceeds the saturation limit in ethanol. Polymerization yields low- to high- molecular weight polymers and, following condensation reaction, particles of 1–2 nm. Then growing of the nuclei occurs following a LaMer growth pattern, until reaching a diameter of 5–7 nm,

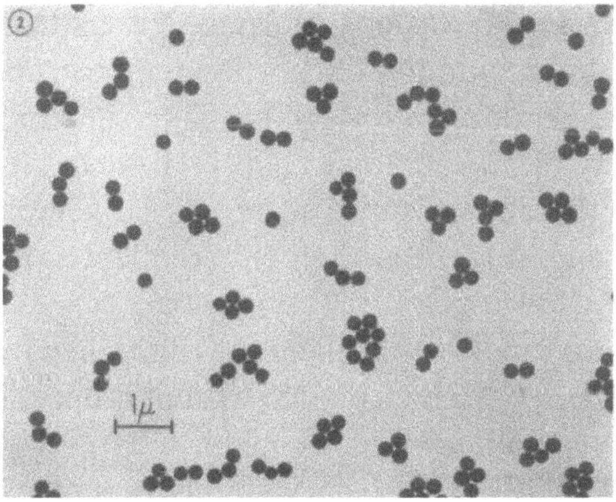

Figure 2.33 TEM image of monodisperse silica NPs synthesized by Stöber protocol [145]. Reproduced from [145] with permission of Elsevier.

that is the critical value after which they begin to aggregate to form silica NPs [146].

In reverse w/o microemulsion, silica precursors are confined inside micelles and the hydrolysis take place in presence of surfactants. One of the major drawbacks of this technique is related to the purification of the product from the surfactants.

Syntheses of spherical silica NPs with finely controlled size dispersion have been reported. Hristov *et al.* reported the synthesis of silica NPs in the range 10–120 nm in aqueous environment and investigated the use of organic solvents with different polarities (ethanol, isopropanol, 1-butanol, 1-hexanol and cyclohexane) in order to control the monomers generation rates and transfer [147].

Quan *et al.* have recently reported the synthetic route and a biomedical application of silica NPs in the range 7–120 nm in which bigger NPs were synthesized by repeated Stöber processes, employing smaller particles for seed-mediated growth [148].

As well as spherical silica NPs, hollow silica nanoshells have been largely investigated either by soft or hard template based syntheses. Zhang *et al.* reported a kinetically controlled template-free synthetic route for monodisperse hollow silica materials with various morphologies, including tubes, crutches, ribbons, bundles and bells, demonstrating the versatility of sol-gel process for synthesizing silica particles with a huge variety of morphologies [149]. However, it is worth to notice that, the size of those materials largely exceeded the nanometer range and, thus, their employment as medical tools is not straightforward.

Silica surface can be easily chemically modified by employing alcoxysilane moieties which bind to silanols groups. The reaction can be achieved both in aqueous media and in organic solvents. Silica coupling with silane-bearing moieties is often carried out in non-aqueous environment to prevent its hydrolysis and condensation and achieve direct coupling with silanols. In particular, aminopropyl triethoxy silane and PEG-silanes are among the most used surface capping agents for silica NPs, providing both full coverage and straightforward anchoring points (*e.g.* amines, thiols and carboxyl groups) for further modifications.

Quantum dots

Semiconductors have deeply revolutionized computer science and electronics from their introduction in the 1950's. Today, reduction of semiconductors sizes up-to nanometer scale has paved the way for their introduction in biological sciences. Indeed, semiconductor NPs, termed quantum dots (QDs), have demonstrated extraordinary optical properties such as strong narrow band luminescence, high quantum yield and high resistance to photobleaching, that allowed them to become the first choice for fluorescent labeling, overwhelming organic molecules. Their size is usually comprised between 2 and 10 nm.

Nowadays, the fine selection of semiconductors has allowed the production of QDs with the desired optical activity. The most diffused semiconductor for the production of QDs is CdSe, whose luminescence wavelength is controlled by size and shape tuning, and its quantum yield is governed by the surface chemistry *i.e.* by the amount of dangling bonds which favor non-radiative decay pathways.

Other typical QDs are composed by InP, CdTe, PbS and PbSe, whose absorption and emission spectra are finely tunable in a broad range of wavelength by size control (Figure 2.34) [150].

The control over the surface chemistry of QDs is required to modulate their emission behavior. One of the most promising approach is related to the development of core-shell QDs, composites by two or more semiconductor materials, such as CdSe/ZnS core/shell QDs. Core/shell QDs can be further modify by capping moieties or by embedding them in oxide layers such as silica.

Wet chemistry routes for the synthesis of QDs have been extensively explored, especially for chalcogenides, for which ternary and even quaternary compounds with extremely accurate control over elemental composition, size and shape have been produced with relatively simple chemical pathways. For example, copper-based chalcogenides multinary QDs with extremely low size dispersion, different crystallographic structure and anisotropic shape (*e.g.* multipods) have been synthesized and are reported in Figure 2.35 [151].

Wet chemical approaches are based on the conventional precursor monomers nucleation and growth, either by w/o microemulsion, hot injection method or ultrasound (or microwave) assisted reductions. However, most of the protocols reported are based on high temperature reactions(Murray) or especially for multinary compounds, QDs are required to be annealed after the synthesis to remove defects derived from lattice mismatches and obtain high quality QDs.

At this regard, it is useful to remind that the parameters which determine QDs quality are the fluorescence quantum yield and the number of cycles of excitation and emission that can be performed preserving their photostability.

Surface modifications of QDs have allowed both their direct synthesis in aqueous environments, and their enhanced biocompatibility. Phosphates, carboxyles and amines have been employed as efficient capping ligands and stabilizers for QDs production in water [152]. Notably, biological moieties such as DNA, peptides,

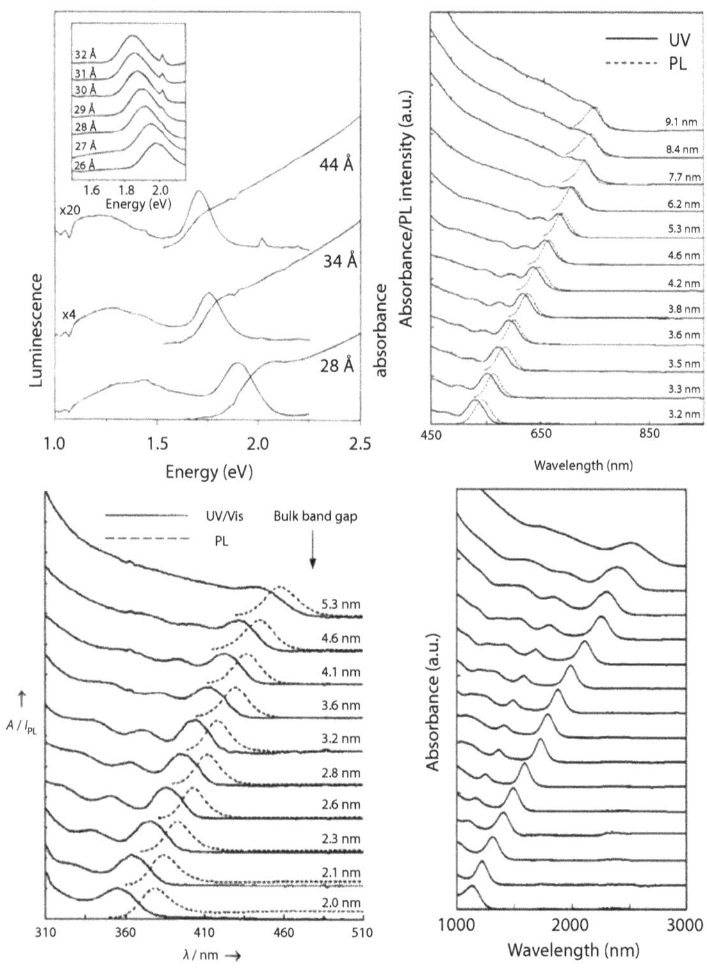

Figure 2.34 Size-dependent optical behavior of (a) InP, (b) CdTe, (c) PbS and (d) PbSe quantum dots. (a) Reproduced from [163] with permission of John Wiley & Sons Inc. (b) Reproduced with permission from [164]. Copyright 2004 American Chemical Society. (c) Reproduced with permission from [165]. Copyright 2003 American Chemical Society. (d) Reproduced with permission from [166]. Copyright 1996 American Chemical Society.

proteins or antibodies have been successfully conjugated to QDs by exploiting standard EDC/NHS couplings [153].

As already reviewed for noble metals, thiols are, among all, the most popular anchoring moiety also for QDs. For example, glutathione has been employed for capping CdSe, CdS,

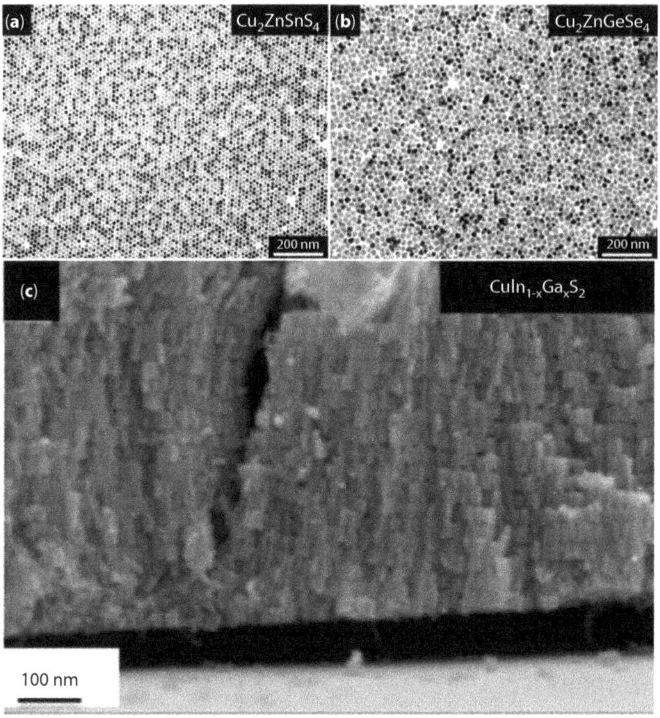

Figure 2.35 TEM images of Cu based quaternary chalcogenides [151]. (a) Reprinted with permission from [167]. Copyright 2013 American Chemical Society. (b) Reprinted with permission from [168]. Copyright 2012 American Chemical Society. (c) Reprinted with permission from [169]. Copyright 2012 American Chemical Society.

and CdTe QDs, acting both as stabilizer and biocompatibility enhancer [154]. Notably, thiolate-capping moieties strongly modified QDs luminescence, either enhancing or suppressing it, depending on their chemical composition [155].

References

1. Roduner, E. Size matters : why nanomaterials are different. *Chem.Soc.Rev.* 583–592, 2006.
2. Roduner, E. *Nanoscopic Materials: Size-Dependent Phenomena* 2006.

3. Luo, S.-N., Strachan, A. & Swift, D. C. Vibrational density of states and Lindemann melting law. *J. Chem. Phys.* 122, 194709, 2005.
4. Gilvarry, J. J. Amplitudes of Thermal Vibration at Fusion. *Phys. Rev.* 103, 1700–1704, 1956.
5. Lai, S. L., Guo, J. Y., Petrova, V., Ramanath, G. & Allen, L. H. Size-Dependent Melting Properties of Small Tin Particles: Nanocalorimetric Measurements. *Phys. Rev. Lett.* 77, 99–102, 1996.
6. McBride, J. R., Dukes, A. D., Schreuder, M. A. & Rosenthal, S. J. On ultrasmall nanocrystals. *Chem. Phys. Lett.* 498, 1–9, 2010.
7. Mei, Q. S. & Lu, K. Melting and superheating of crystalline solids: From bulk to nanocrystals. *Prog. Mater. Sci.* 52, 1175–1262, 2007.
8. Daeges, J., Gleiter, H. & Perepezko, J. H. Superheating of metal crystals. *Phys. Lett. A* 119, 79–82, 1986.
9. Shi, Z., Wynblatt, P. & Srinivasan, S.. Melting behavior of nanosized lead particles embedded in an aluminum matrix. *Acta Mater.* 52, 2305–2316, 2004.
10. Saka, H., Nishikawa, Y. & Imura, T. Melting temperature of In particles embedded in an Al matrix. *Philos. Mag. A* 57, 895–906, 1988.
11. Noguez, C. Surface Plasmons on Metal Nanoparticles: The Influence of Shape and Physical Environment. *J. Phys. Chem. C* 111, 3806–3819, 2007.
12. Zhang, J. Z. & Noguez, C. Plasmonic optical properties and applications of metal nanostructures. *Plasmonics* 3, 127–150, 2008.
13. Pastoriza-Santos, I. & Liz-Marzán, L. M. Colloidal silver nanoplates. State of the art and future challenges. *J. Mater. Chem.* 18, 1724, 2008.
14. Huang, X., Neretina, S. & El-Sayed, M. A. Gold nanorods: From synthesis and properties to biological and biomedical applications. *Adv. Mater.* 21, 4880–4910, 2009.
15. Buceta, D., Piñeiro, Y., Vázquez-Vázquez, C., Rivas, J. & López-Quintela, M. Metallic Clusters: Theoretical Background, Properties and Synthesis in Microemulsions. *Catalysts* 4, 356–374, 2014.
16. Chris I. Richards, Sungmoon Choi, Jung-Cheng Hsiang, Yasuko Antoku, Tom Vosch, Angelo Bongiorno, Yih-Ling Tzeng, and Robert M. Dickson, Oligonucleotide-Stabilized Ag Nanocluster Fluorophores. Journal of the American Chemical Society 130 (15), 5038–5039, 2008.

17. Chen, L.-Y., Wang, C.-W., Yuan, Z. & Chang, H. Fluorescent gold nanoclusters: recent advances in sensing and imaging. *Anal. Chem.* 87, 216–29, 2015.
18. Kittel, C. *Introduction to Solid State Physics.* (John Wiley & Sons, Inc., 1986).
19. Weidman, M. C., Beck, M. E., Hoffman, R. S., Prins, F. & Tisdale, W. A. Monodisperse, Air-Stable PbS Nanocrystals via Precursor Stoichiometry Control. *ACS Nano* 8, 6363–6371, 2014.
20. Pietryga, J.M., Schaller, R.D., Werder, D., Stewart, M.H., Klimov, V.I. and Hollingsworth, J.A. *Journal of the American Chemical Society* 126 (38), 11752–11753, 2004.
21. Sorensen, C. M. *Cap. 6: Magnetism Nanoscale Materials in Chemistry.* 83, 2002.
22. Cullity, B. D. & Graham, C. D. *Introduction to Magnetic Materials.* John Wiley & Sons, Inc., 2009.
23. Mørup, S. & Hansen, M. F. Superparamagnetic Particles in *Handbook of Magnetism and Advanced Magnetic Materials,* John Wiley & Sons, Ltd, 2007.
24. Angappane, S., Park, J., Jang, Y., Hyeon, T. & Park, J.-G. Magnetic Pd nanoparticles: effects of surface atoms. *J. Phys. Condens. Matter* 20, 295209, 2008.
25. Nealon, G. L. *et al.* Magnetism in gold nanoparticles. *Nanoscale* 4, 5244, 2012.
26. Li, C. Y. *et al.* Intrinsic magnetic moments of gold nanoparticles. *Phys. Rev. B – Condens. Matter Mater. Phys.* **83**, 2011.
27. Hong, G., Diao, S., Antaris, A. L. & Dai, H. Carbon Nanomaterials for Biological Imaging and Nanomedicinal Therapy. *Chem. Rev.* 115, 10816–10906, 2015.
28. Kroto, H. W., Heath, J. R., O'Brien, S. C., Curl, R. F. & Smalley, R. E. C60: Buckminsterfullerene. *Nature* 318, 162–163, 1985.
29. Partha, R. & Conyers, J. L. Biomedical applications of functionalized fullerene-based nanomaterials. *Int. J. Nanomedicine* 4, 261–275, 2009.
30. Smith, A. M., Mancini, M. C. & Nie, S. Second window for *in vivo* imaging. *Nat. Nanotechnol.* 4, 710–711, 2009.
31. Maestro, L. M. *et al.* Heating efficiency of multi-walled carbon nanotubes in the first and second biological windows. *Nanoscale* 5, 7882, 2013.

32. Harrison, B. S. & Atala, A. Carbon nanotube applications for tissue engineering. *Biomaterials* 28, 344–353, 2007.
33. Novoselov, K. S. *et al.* Electric field in atomically thin carbon films. *Science (80-.).* 306, 666–669, 2004.
34. Spirito, D. *et al.* High performance bilayer-graphene terahertz detectors. *Appl. Phys. Lett.* 104, 61111, 2014.
35. Kuila, T. *et al.* Recent advances in graphene-based biosensors. *Biosens. Bioelectron.* 26, 4637–4648, 2011.
36. Wu, L., Chu, H. S., Koh, W. S. & Li, E. P. Highly sensitive graphene biosensors based on surface plasmon resonance. *Opt. Express* 18, 14395, 2010.
37. Chung, C. *et al.* Biomedical Applications of Graphene and Graphene Oxide. *Acc. Chem. Res.* 46, 2211–2224, 2013.
38. Zhu, S. *et al.* The photoluminescence mechanism in carbon dots (graphene quantum dots, carbon nanodots, and polymer dots): current state and future perspective. *Nano Res.* 8, 355–381, 2015.
39. Zheng, X. T., Ananthanarayanan, A., Luo, K. Q. & Chen, P. Glowing Graphene Quantum Dots and Carbon Dots: Properties, Syntheses, and Biological Applications. *Small* 11, 1620–1636, 2015.
40. Mochalin, V. N., Shenderova, O., Ho, D. & Gogotsi, Y. The properties and applications of nanodiamonds. *Nat. Nanotechnol.* 7, 11–23, 2012.
41. Chen, R. J. *et al.* Noncovalent functionalization of carbon nanotubes for highly specific electronic biosensors. *Proc. Natl. Acad. Sci.* 100, 4984–4989, 2003.
42. Shim, M., Shi Kam, N. W., Chen, R. J., Li, Y. & Dai, H. Functionalization of Carbon Nanotubes for Biocompatibility and Biomolecular Recognition. *Nano Lett.* 2, 285–288, 2002.
43. Hirsch, A. Functionalization of Single-Walled Carbon Nanotubes. *Angew. Chemie Int. Ed.* 41, 1853, 2002.
44. Georgakilas, V. *et al.* Organic Functionalization of Carbon Nanotubes. *J. Am. Chem. Soc.* 124, 760–761, 2002.
45. Dyke, C. A. & Tour, J. M. Covalent Functionalization of Single-Walled Carbon Nanotubes for Materials Applications. *J. Phys. Chem. A* 108, 11151–11159, 2004.
46. Akbarzadeh, A. *et al.* Liposome: classification, preparation, and applications. *Nanoscale Res. Lett.* 8, 102, 2013.

47. Laouini, A. *et al.* Preparation, Characterization and Applications of Liposomes: State of the Art. *J. Colloid Sci. Biotechnol.* 1, 147–168, 2012.
48. Bangham, A. D. Liposomes: the Babraham connection. *Chem. Phys. Lipids* 64, 275–285, 1993.
49. Patil, Y. P. & Jadhav, S. Novel methods for liposome preparation. *Chem. Phys. Lipids* 177, 8–18, 2014.
50. Woodle, M. C. & Papahadjopoulos, D. Liposome preparation and size characterization, *Methods in Enzymology* 171, pp. 193–217, 1989.
51. Costa, A. P., Xu, X. & Burgess, D. J. Freeze-anneal-thaw cycling of unilamellar liposomes: Effect on encapsulation efficiency. *Pharm. Res.* 31, 97–103, 2014.
52. Huang, Z. *et al.* Progress involving new techniques for liposome preparation. *Asian J. Pharm. Sci.* 9, 176–182, 2014.
53. Mali, A. D. & Bathe, R. S. An Updated Review on Liposome Drug Delivery System. *Asian J. Pharm. Res.* 5, 151, 2015.
54. Koynova, R. & Tenchov, B. Recent Progress in Liposome Production, Relevance to Drug Delivery and Nanomedicine. *Recent Pat. Nanotechnol.* 9, 86–93, 2015.
55. Elhissi, A., Phoenix, D. & Ahmed, W. in *Emerging Nanotechnologies for Manufacturing, Emerging Nanotechnologies for Manufacturing,* pp. 402–417 Elsevier, 2015.
56. Gupta, V. & Nayak, S. Dendrimers: A Review on Synthetic Approaches. *J. Appl. Pharm. Sci.* 117–122, 2015.
57. Hsu, H. J., Bugno, J., Lee, S. R. & Hong, S. Dendrimer-based nanocarriers: a versatile platform for drug delivery. *Wiley Interdiscip. Rev. Nanomedicine Nanobiotechnology* 9, 1–21, 2017.
58. Duncan, R. & Izzo, L. Dendrimer biocompatibility and toxicity. *Adv. Drug Deliv. Rev.* 57, 2215–2237, 2005.
59. Jain, K., Kesharwani, P., Gupta, U. & Jain, N. K. Dendrimer toxicity: Let's meet the challenge. *Int. J. Pharm.* 394, 122–142, 2010.
60. Torchilin, V. in *Multifunctional Pharmaceutical Nanocarriers* 1–32, 2008.
61. Liu, Z., Jiao, Y., Wang, Y., Zhou, C. & Zhang, Z. Polysaccharides-based nanoparticles as drug delivery systems. *Adv. Drug Deliv. Rev.* 60, 1650–1662, 2008.

62. Swierczewska, M., Han, H. S., Kim, K., Park, J. H. & Lee, S. Polysaccharide-based nanoparticles for theranostic nanomedicine. *Adv. Drug Deliv. Rev.* 99, 70–84, 2016.
63. Grenha, A. Chitosan nanoparticles: A survey of preparation methods. *J. Drug Target.* 20, 291–300, 2012.
64. Landriscina, A., Rosen, J. & Friedman, A. J. Biodegradable chitosan nanoparticles in drug delivery for infectious disease. *Nanomedicine* 10, 1609–1619, 2015.
65. Lemarchand, C., Gref, R. & Couvreur, P. Polysaccharide-decorated nanoparticles. *Eur. J. Pharm. Biopharm.* 58, 327–341, 2004.
66. Berry, C. C., Wells, S., Charles, S., Aitchison, G. & Curtis, A. S. G. Cell response to dextran-derivatised iron oxide nanoparticles post internalisation. *Biomaterials* 25, 5405–5413, 2004.
67. Iakobson, O. D., Dobrodumov, A. V., Saprykina, N. N. & Shevchenko, N. N. Dextran Nanoparticles Cross-Linked in Aqueous and Aqueous/Alcoholic Media. *Macromol. Chem. Phys.* 218, 1600523, 2017.
68. Ganesh, S., Iyer, A. K., Morrissey, D. V. & Amiji, M. M. Hyaluronic acid based self-assembling nanosystems for CD44 target mediated siRNA delivery to solid tumors. *Biomaterials* 34, 3489–3502, 2013.
69. Choi, K. Y. *et al.* Self-assembled hyaluronic acid nanoparticles for active tumor targeting. *Biomaterials* 31, 106–114, 2010.
70. Swann, D. A. *et al.* Role of hyaluronic acid in joint lubrication. *Ann. Rheum. Dis.* 33, 318–326, 1974.
71. Voigt, J. & Driver, V. R. Hyaluronic acid derivatives and their healing effect on burns, epithelial surgical wounds, and chronic wounds: A systematic review and meta-analysis of randomized controlled trials. *Wound Repair Regen.* 20, 317–331, 2012.
72. Cai, S., Xie, Y., Bagby, T. R., Cohen, M. S. & Forrest, M. L. Intralymphatic Chemotherapy Using a Hyaluronan–Cisplatin Conjugate. *J. Surg. Res.* 147, 247–252, 2008.
73. Lee, H., Lee, K. & Park, T. G. Hyaluronic Acid–Paclitaxel Conjugate Micelles: Synthesis, Characterization, and Antitumor Activity. *Bioconjug. Chem.* 19, 1319–1325, 2008.
74. Camacho, K. M. *et al.* Synergistic antitumor activity of camptothecin–doxorubicin combinations and their conjugates with hyaluronic acid. *J. Control. Release* 210, 198–207, 2015.

75. Ferguson, E. L., Alshame, A. M. J. & Thomas, D. W. Evaluation of hyaluronic acid–protein conjugates for polymer masked–unmasked protein therapy. *Int. J. Pharm.* 402, 95–102, 2010.
76. Li, N. *et al.* Polysaccharide-Gold Nanocluster Supramolecular Conjugates as a Versatile Platform for the Targeted Delivery of Anticancer Drugs. *Sci. Rep.* 4, 4164, 2015.
77. Danhier, F. *et al.* PLGA-based nanoparticles: An overview of biomedical applications. *J. Control. Release* 161, 505–522, 2012.
78. Yu, J. *et al.* Electrospun PLGA Fibers Incorporated with Functionalized Biomolecules for Cardiac Tissue Engineering. *Tissue Eng. Part A* 20, 1896–1907, 2014.
79. Liu, R. *et al.* Effects of the molecular weight of PLGA on degradation and drug release *in vitro* from an mPEG-PLGA nanocarrier. *Chem. Res. Chinese Univ.* 32, 848–853, 2016.
80. Astete, C. E. & Sabliov, C. M. Synthesis and characterization of PLGA nanoparticles. *J. Biomater. Sci. Polym. Ed.* 17, 247–289, 2006.
81. Thomasin, C., Nam-Trân, H., Merkle, H. P. & Gander, B. Drug Microencapsulation by PLA/PLGA Coacervation in the Light of Thermodynamics. 1. Overview and Theoretical Considerations. *J. Pharm. Sci.* 87, 259–268, 1998.
82. Miladi, K., Sfar, S., Fessi, H. & Elaissari, A. in *Polymer Nanoparticles for Nanomedicines* 17–53, Springer International Publishing, 2016.
83. Lunov, O. *et al.* Amino-Functionalized Polystyrene Nanoparticles Activate the NLRP3 Inflammasome in Human Macrophages. *ACS Nano* 5, 9648–9657, 2011.
84. Tenzer, S. *et al.* Rapid formation of plasma protein corona critically affects nanoparticle pathophysiology. *Nat. Nanotechnol.* 8, 772–781, 2013.
85. Milošević, I. *et al.* Synthesis and size control of polystyrene nanoparticles via 'liquid crystalline' nanoemulsion. *Microporous Mesoporous Mater.* 120, 7–11, 2009.
86. Pargen, S., Willems, C., Keul, H., Pich, A. & Möller, M. Surfactant-Free Synthesis of Polystyrene Nanoparticles Using Oligoglycidol Macromonomers. *Macromolecules* 45, 1230–1240, 2012.
87. Kim, M. S. *et al.* Synthesis of polystyrene nanoparticles with monodisperse size distribution and positive surface charge using metal stearates. *Macromol. Res.* 16, 178–181, 2008.

88. Yang, Y. *et al.* Biodegradation and Mineralization of Polystyrene by Plastic-Eating Mealworms: Part 2. Role of Gut Microorganisms. *Environ. Sci. Technol.* 49, 12087–12093, 2015.
89. Turkevich, J., Stevenson, P. C. & Hillier, J. A study of the nucleation and growth processes in the synthesis of colloidal gold. *Discuss. Faraday Soc.* 11, 55, 1951.
90. LaMer, V. K. & Dinegar, R. H. Theory, Production and Mechanism of Formation of Monodispersed Hydrosols. *J. Am. Chem. Soc.* 72, 4847–4854, 1950.
91. Piella, J., Bastús, N. G. & Puntes, V. Size-Controlled Synthesis of Sub-10-nanometer Citrate-Stabilized Gold Nanoparticles and Related Optical Properties. *Chem. Mater.* 28, 1066–1075, 2016.
92. Bastús, N. G., Comenge, J. & Puntes, V. Kinetically controlled seeded growth synthesis of citrate-stabilized gold nanoparticles of up to 200 nm: Size focusing versus ostwald ripening. *Langmuir* 27, 11098–11105, 2011.
93. Li, N., Zhao, P. & Astruc, D. Anisotropic gold nanoparticles: Synthesis, properties, applications, and toxicity. *Angew. Chemie - Int. Ed.* 53, 1756–1789, 2014.
94. Scarabelli, L., Sánchez-Iglesias, A., Pérez-Juste, J. & Liz-Marzán, L. M. A 'Tips and Tricks' Practical Guide to the Synthesis of Gold Nanorods. *J. Phys. Chem. Lett.* 6, 4270–4279, 2015.
95. Pérez-Juste, J., Pastoriza-Santos, I., Liz-Marzán, L. M. & Mulvaney, P. Gold nanorods: Synthesis, characterization and applications. *Coord. Chem. Rev.* 249, 1870–1901, 2005.
96. Tong, W., Walsh, M. J., Mulvaney, P., Etheridge, J. & Funston, A. M. Control of Symmetry Breaking Size and Aspect Ratio in Gold Nanorods: Underlying Role of Silver Nitrate. *J. Phys. Chem. C* 121, 3549–3559, 2017.
97. Hubert, F., Testard, F. & Spalla, O. Cetyltrimethylammonium Bromide Silver Bromide Complex as the Capping Agent of Gold Nanorods. *Langmuir* 24, 9219–9222, 2008.
98. Pallavicini, P. *et al.* Triton X-100 for three-plasmon gold nanostars with two photothermally active NIR (near IR) and SWIR (short-wavelength IR) channels. *Chem. Commun.* 49, 6265, 2013.
99. Shi, W., Sahoo, Y., Swihart, M. T. & Prasad, P. N. Gold Nanoshells on Polystyrene Cores for Control of Surface Plasmon Resonance. *Langmuir* 21, 1610–1617, 2005.

100. Guan, Y., Xue, Z., Liang, J., Huang, Z. & Yang, W. One-pot synthesis of size-tunable hollow gold nanoshells via APTES-in-water suspension. *Colloids Surfaces A Physicochem. Eng. Asp.* 502, 6–12, 2016.
101. Porel, S., Singh, S. & Radhakrishnan, T. P. Polygonal gold nanoplates in a polymer matrix. *Chem. Commun. Camb.* 2387–2389, 2005.
102. Chen, L. *et al.* High-yield seedless synthesis of triangular gold nanoplates through oxidative etching. *Nano Lett.* 14, 7201–7206, 2014.
103. Jadhav, S. A. Functional self-assembled monolayers (SAMs) of organic compounds on gold nanoparticles. *J. Mater. Chem.* 22, 5894, 2012.
104. Voliani, V., Luin, S., Ricci, F. & Beltram, F. Single-step bifunctional coating for selectively conjugable nanoparticles. *Nanoscale* 2, 2783–2789, 2010.
105. Voliani, V., Ricci, F., Luin, S. & Beltram, F. Peptidic coating for gold nanospheres multifunctionalizable with photostable and photolabile moieties. *J. Mater. Chem.* 22, 14487, 2012.
106. Shirtcliffe, N., Nickel, U. & Schneider, S. Reproducible Preparation of Silver Sols with Small Particle Size Using Borohydride Reduction: For Use as Nuclei for Preparation of Larger Particles. *J. Colloid Interface Sci.* 211, 122–129, 1999.
107. Pillai, Z. S. & Kamat, P. V. What Factors Control the Size and Shape of Silver Nanoparticles in the Citrate Ion Reduction Method? *J. Phys. Chem. B* 108, 945–951, 2004.
108. Nair, L. S. & Laurencin, C. T. Silver Nanoparticles: Synthesis and Therapeutic Applications. *J. Biomed. Nanotechnol.* 3, 301–316, 2007.
109. Agnihotri, S., Mukherji, S. & Mukherji, S. Size-controlled silver nanoparticles synthesized over the range 5–100 nm using the same protocol and their antibacterial efficacy. *RSC Adv.* 4, 3974–3983, 2014.
110. Rainville, L., Dorais, M.-C. & Boudreau, D. Controlled synthesis of low polydispersity Ag@SiO2 core–shell nanoparticles for use in plasmonic applications. *RSC Adv.* 3, 13953, 2013.
111. Bastús, N. G., Merkoçi, F., Piella, J. & Puntes, V. Synthesis of Highly Monodisperse Citrate-Stabilized Silver Nanoparticles

of up to 200 nm: Kinetic Control and Catalytic Properties. *Chem. Mater.* 26, 2836–2846, 2014.
112. Garcia-Leis, A., Garcia-Ramos, J. V. & Sanchez-Cortes, S. Silver nanostars with high SERS performance. *J. Phys. Chem. C* 117, 7791–7795, 2013.
113. Guoli Si, Wentao Shi, Kai Li, Zhanfang Ma, Synthesis of PSS-capped triangular silver nanoplates with tunable SPR. *Colloids and Surfaces A: Physicochemical and Engineering Aspects* 380, 257–260, 2011.
114. Lee, G. P. *et al.* The Light Driven Transformation Processes of Anisotropic Silver Nanoparticles. *ACS Nano* 7: 5911–5921, 2013.
115. Silver, P., Pietrobon, B., Mceachran, M. & Kitaev, V. Synthesis of Size-Controlled Faceted Tunable Plasmonic Properties and Self- Assembly of These Nanorods. *ACS Nano* 3, 21–26, 2009.
116. Mahmoud, M. A. & El-sayed, M. a. Different Plasmon Sensing Behavior of Silver and Gold Nanorods. *Phys. Chem.* 4(9): 1541–1545, 2013.
117. Kang, H. *et al.* One-step synthesis of silver nanoshells with bumps for highly sensitive near-IR SERS nanoprobes. *J. Mater. Chem. B* 2, 4415, 2014.
118. Bashouti, M. Y. *et al.* Functionalization of Silver Nanowires Surface using Ag-C Bonds in a Sequential Reductive Method. *ACS Appl. Mater. Interfaces* 7, 21657–21661, 2015.
119. Islam, A., Anwarul Kabir Bhuiya, M. & Saidul Islam, M. A Review on Chemical Synthesis Process of Platinum Nanoparticles. *Asia Pacific J. Energy Environ.* 1, 107, 2014.
120. Bigall, N. C. *et al.* Monodisperse platinum nanospheres with adjustable diameters from 10 to 100 nm: Synthesis and distinct optical properties. *Nano Lett.* 8, 4588–4592, 2008.
121. Song, H., Kim, F., Connor, S., Somorjai, G. A. & Yang, P. Pt Nanocrystals: Shape Control and Langmuir–Blodgett Monolayer Formation. *J. Phys. Chem. B* 109, 188–193, 2005.
122. Long, N. V. *et al.* The synthesis and characterization of platinum nanoparticles: a method of controlling the size and morphology. *Nanotechnology* 21, 35605, 2010.
123. Teng, X. & Yang, H. Synthesis of Platinum Multipods: An Induced Anisotropic Growth. *Nano Lett.* 5, 885–891, 2005.

124. Chen, J., Herricks, T., Geissler, M. & Xia, Y. Single-Crystal Nanowires of Platinum Can Be Synthesized by Controlling the Reaction Rate of a Polyol Process. *J. Am. Chem. Soc.* 126, 10854–10855, 2004.
125. Pedone, D., Moglianetti, M., De Luca, E., Bardi, G. & Pompa, P. P. Platinum nanoparticles in nanobiomedicine. *Chem. Soc. Rev.* 46, 4951–4975, 2017.
126. Gawande, M. B. *et al.* Cu and Cu-Based Nanoparticles: Synthesis and Applications in Catalysis. *Chem. Rev.* 116, 3722–3811, 2016.
127. Dang, T. M. D., Le, T. T. T., Fribourg-Blanc, E. & Dang, M. C. Synthesis and optical properties of copper nanoparticles prepared by a chemical reduction method. *Adv. Nat. Sci. Nanosci. Nanotechnol.* 2, 15009, 2011.
128. Duggan, J. N., Bozack, M. J. & Roberts, C. B. The synthesis and arrested oxidation of amorphous cobalt nanoparticles using DMSO as a functional solvent. *J. Nanoparticle Res.* 15,, 2013.
129. Oyarzún, S., Tamion, A., Tournus, F., Dupuis, V. & Hillenkamp, M. Size effects in the magnetic anisotropy of embedded cobalt nanoparticles: from shape to surface. *Sci. Rep.* 5, 14749, 2015.
130. Meziane, L. *et al.* Hcp cobalt nanocrystals with high magnetic anisotropy prepared by easy one-pot synthesis. *Nanoscale* 8, 18640–18645, 2016.
131. Srikala, D., Singh, V. N., Banerjee, A., Mehta, B. R. & Patnaik, S. Control of magnetism in cobalt nanoparticles by oxygen passivation. *J. Phys. Chem. C* 112, 13882–13885, 2008.
132. Ekinci, Y., Solak, H. H. & Löffler, J. F. Plasmon resonances of aluminum nanoparticles and nanorods. *J. Appl. Phys.* 104, 2008.
133. Sugawa, K. *et al.* Refractive index susceptibility of the plasmonic palladium nanoparticle: Potential as the third plasmonic sensing material. *ACS Nano* 9, 1895–1904, 2015.
134. Watson, A. M. *et al.* Rhodium nanoparticles for ultraviolet plasmonics. *Nano Lett.* 15, 1095–1100, 2015.
135. Chen, J. *et al.* Plasmonic nickel nanoantennas. *Small* 7, 2341–2347, 2011.
136. Niederberger, M. *et al.* Nonaqueous Synthesis of Metal Oxide Nanoparticles: Review and Indium Oxide as Case Study for the Dependence of Particle Morphology on Precursors and Solvents. *ChemInform* 38,, 2007.

137. Pinna, N. & Niederberger, M. Surfactant-free nonaqueous synthesis of metal oxide nanostructures. *Angew. Chemie - Int. Ed.* 47, 5292–5304, 2008.
138. Djerdj, I., Arčon, D., Jagličić, Z. & Niederberger, M. Nonaqueous synthesis of metal oxide nanoparticles: Short review and doped titanium dioxide as case study for the preparation of transition metal-doped oxide nanoparticles. *J. Solid State Chem.* 181, 1571–1581, 2008.
139. Wu, W., Wu, Z., Yu, T., Jiang, C. & Kim, W.-S. Recent progress on magnetic iron oxide nanoparticles: synthesis, surface functional strategies and biomedical applications. *Sci. Technol. Adv. Mater.* 16, 23501, 2015.
140. Hyeon, T., Lee, S. S., Park, J., Chung, Y. & Na, H. Bin. Synthesis of Highly Crystalline and Monodisperse Maghemite Nanocrystallites without a Size-Selection Process. *J. Am. Chem. Soc.* 123, 12798–12801, 2001.
141. Zhou, Z. *et al.* Anisotropic shaped iron oxide nanostructures: Controlled synthesis and proton relaxation shortening effects. *Chem. Mater.* 27, 3505–3515, 2015.
142. Boni, A., Albertazzi, L., Innocenti, C., Gemmi, M. & Bifone, A. Water Dispersal and Functionalization of Hydrophobic Iron Oxide Nanoparticles with Lipid-Modified Poly(amidoamine) Dendrimers. *Langmuir* 29, 10973–10979, 2013.
143. Liang, C.-H. *et al.* Iron Oxide/Gold Core/Shell Nanoparticles for Ultrasensitive Detection of Carbohydrate–Protein Interactions. *Anal. Chem.* 81, 7750–7756, 2009.
144. Wang, L. *et al.* Iron oxide–gold core–shell nanoparticles and thin film assembly. *J. Mater. Chem.* 15, 1821, 2005.
145. Stöber, W., Fink, A. & Bohn, E. Controlled growth of monodisperse silica spheres in the micron size range. *J. Colloid Interface Sci.* 26, 62–69, 1968.
146. Masalov, V. M., Sukhinina, N. S., Kudrenko, E. A. & Emelchenko, G. A. Mechanism of formation and nanostructure of Stöber silica particles. *Nanotechnology* 22, 275718, 2011.
147. Hristov, D. R., Mahon, E. & Dawson, K. A. Controlling aqueous silica nanoparticle synthesis in the 10–100 nm range. *Chem. Commun.* 51, 17420–17423, 2015.

148. Quan, B., Lee, C., Yoo, J. S. & Piao, Y. Facile scalable synthesis of highly monodisperse small silica nanoparticles using alkaline buffer solution and their application for efficient sentinel lymph node mapping. *J. Mater. Chem. B* 5, 586–594, 2017.
149. Zhang, A.-Q., Li, H.-J., Qian, D.-J. & Chen, M. Kinetically-controlled template-free synthesis of hollow silica micro-/Nanostructures with unusual morphologies. *Nanotechnology* 25, 135608, 2014.
150. Michalet, X. *et al.* Quantum dots for live cells, *in vivo* imaging, and diagnostics. *Science (80-.).* 307, 538–544, 2005.
151. Kovalenko, M. V. *et al.* Prospects of Nanoscience with Nanocrystals. *ACS Nano* 9, 1012–1057, 2015.
152. Zhang, Y. & Clapp, A. Overview of Stabilizing Ligands for Biocompatible Quantum Dot Nanocrystals. *Sensors* 11, 11036–11055, 2011.
153. Boeneman, K. *et al.* Quantum Dot DNA Bioconjugates: Attachment Chemistry Strongly Influences the Resulting Composite Architecture. *ACS Nano* 4, 7253–7266, 2010.
154. Liu, Y.-F. & Yu, J.-S. Selective synthesis of CdTe and high luminescence CdTe/CdS quantum dots: The effect of ligands. *J. Colloid Interface Sci.* 333, 690–698, 2009.
155. Wuister, S. F., de Mello Donegá, C. & Meijerink, A. Influence of Thiol Capping on the Exciton Luminescence and Decay Kinetics of CdTe and CdSe Quantum Dots. *J. Phys. Chem. B* 108, 17393–17397, 2004.
156. Koray Yurekli, Cynthia A. Mitchell, and Ramanan Krishnamoorti. Small-Angle Neutron Scattering from Surfactant-Assisted Aqueous Dispersions of Carbon Nanotubes. *Journal of the American Chemical Society* 126 (32), 9902–9903, 2004.
157. L. Zhang, L. Laug, W. Münchgesang, E. Pippel, U. Gösele, M. Brandsch and M. Knez, *Nano Lett.*, 10, 219–223, 2010.
158. W. Zhou, J. Wu and H. Yang, *Nano Lett.*, 13, 2870–2874, 2013.
159. J. Gao, G. Liang, J. S. Cheung, Y. Pan, Y. Kuang, F. Zhao, B. Zhang, X. Zhang, E. X. Wu and B. Xu, *J. Am. Chem. Soc.*, 130, 11828–11833, 2008.
160. M. Moglianetti, E. De Luca, D. Pedone, R. Marotta, T. Catelani, B. Sartori, H. Amenitsch, S. F. Retta and P. P. Pompa, *Nanoscale*, 8, 3739–3752, 2016.

161. C. Xu, Z. Yuan, N. Kohler, J. Kim, M. A. Chung and S. Sun, *J. Am. Chem. Soc.*, 131, 15346–15351, 2009.
162. Y. Xiong, B. J. Wiley and Y. Xia, Angew. Chem., *Int. Ed.*, 46, 7157–7159, 2007.
163. Yu, W. W. and Peng, X. Formation of High-Quality CdS and Other II–VI Semiconductor Nanocrystals in Noncoordinating Solvents: Tunable Reactivity of Monomers. *Angewandte Chemie International Edition*, 41: 2368–2371, 2002.
164. William W. Yu,Joshua C. Falkner,Bertram S. Shih, and, and Vicki L. Colvin, Preparation and Characterization of Monodisperse PbSe Semiconductor Nanocrystals in a Noncoordinating Solvent. *Chemistry of Materials* 16 (17), 3318–3322, 2004.
165. W. William Yu,Y. Andrew Wang, and, and Xiaogang Peng, Formation and Stability of Size-, Shape-, and Structure-Controlled CdTe Nanocrystals: Ligand Effects on Monomers and Nanocrystals. *Chemistry of Materials* 15 (22), 4300–4308, 2003.
166. A. A. Guzelian,J. E. B. Katari,A. V. Kadavanich,U. Banin,K. Hamad,E. Juban, and, A. P. Alivisatos, R. H. Wolters,C. C. Arnold, and, and J. R. Heath, Synthesis of Size-Selected, Surface-Passivated InP Nanocrystals. *The Journal of Physical Chemistry* 100 (17), 7212–7219, 1996.
167. Xuelian Yu, Alexey Shavel, Xiaoqiang An, Zhishan Luo, Maria Ibáñez, and Andreu Cabot, Cu2ZnSnS4-Pt and Cu2ZnSnS4-Au Heterostructured Nanoparticles for Photocatalytic Water Splitting and Pollutant Degradation. *Journal of the American Chemical Society* 136 (26), 9236–9239, 2014.
168. Maria Ibáñez, Reza Zamani, Aaron LaLonde, Doris Cadavid, Wenhua Li, Alexey Shavel, Jordi Arbiol, Joan Ramon Morante, Stéphane Gorsse, G. Jeffrey Snyder, and Andreu Cabot, Cu2ZnGeSe4 Nanocrystals: Synthesis and Thermoelectric Properties. *Journal of the American Chemical Society* 134 (9), 4060–4063, 2012.
169. Ajay Singh, Claudia Coughlan, Fathima Laffir, and Kevin M. Ryan, Assembly of CuIn1-xGaxS2 Nanorods into Highly Ordered 2D and 3D Superstructures. *ACS Nano* 6 (8), 6977–6983, 2012
170. Teranishi, T., Hosoe, M., Tanaka, T. and Miyake, M. Size Control of Monodispersed Pt Nanoparticles and Their 2D Organization by Electrophoretic Deposition. *J. Phys. Chem. B.* 103 (19), 3818–3827, 1999.

3

Promising Applications in Medicine

Detecting diseases at an early stage and providing a suitable treatment plan is a major challenge in healthcare to enhance patients' benefits. Development of techniques such as X-ray imaging, NMR, PET and ultrasonography have deeply revolutionized diagnostics, pushing towards non-invasive clinical examinations for diagnoses and disease localization. However, some of these techniques can results in adverse effect, while others are not enough accurate. As an example, imaging techniques based on ionizing radiation can induce damages to fundamental biological macromolecules, such as break in DNA double-strand, resulting in a series of disorders, including cancer. Thus, many efforts are devoted to engineering novel contrast agents, which can provide enhanced diagnostic efficiency with lower radiation doses.

On the other hand, whilst cancer treatments such as chemotherapy or radiotherapy have given renewed hope to oncological patients, the inherent lack of specificity of these techniques is the main cause of the onset of painful side effects and of the reoccurrence of the disease.

The advent of nanotechnology holds the great promise to address these issues. Furthermore, nanomaterials are appealing for combining diagnostics and therapeutics moieties on the same platform (*i.e.*, theranostics). Theranostic agents are all-in-one nanoplatforms that can simultaneously deliver imaging and therapeutic agents to specific sites or organs, enabling detection and treatment of diseases in a single procedure and, thus, improving the patient outcome.

In this chapter, the advances on cancer treatments driven by smart nanomaterials are presented and comprehensively discussed.

3.1 Diagnostics

3.1.1 X-Ray Computed Tomography

X-ray Computed Tomography (CT) is among the most diffused and frequently employed imaging techniques in clinics. It is a quick and non-invasive diagnostic technique which allows for high resolution 3D imaging of large tissues, up to full-body. In CT imaging, the X-ray source and the detector rotate around the patient creating two-dimensional projections of X-rays attenuation through the body, which are then reconstructed by mathematical algorithms to produce a 3D rendering.

X-rays based imaging techniques, in general, rely on the attenuation of X-ray photons while passing through an object, depending linearly on its density and on the fourth power of the atomic number [1]. Photons are attenuated upon interacting with a medium by Rayleigh scattering, pair production, photoelectric effect and Compton scattering. However, photoelectric effect (Figure 3.1) is the dominant source of attenuation for the photon energies commonly used in X-ray diagnostics (30–150 keV).

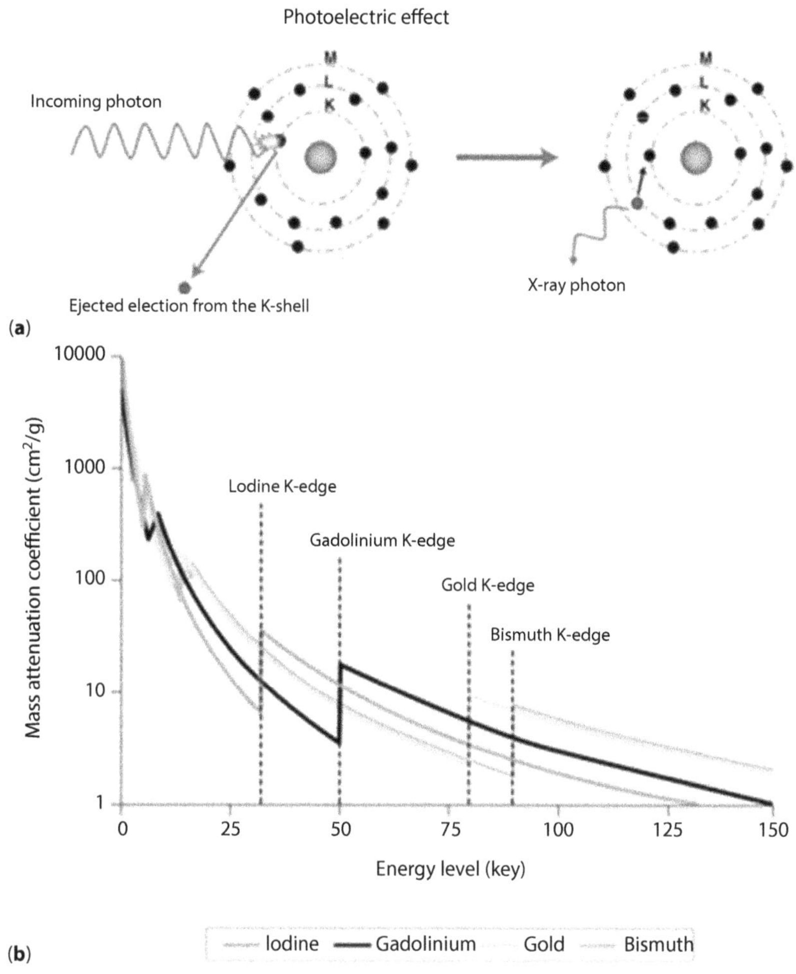

Figure 3.1 Scheme of photoelectric effect followed by emission of an X-ray photon (a) and attenuation coefficients of typical X-ray contrast agents in the range 0–150 keV (b) [2]. Reprinted from [2] with permission of Elsevier.

Hence, we will briefly describe this physical phenomenon and its relevance in X-ray based diagnostics.

In the photoelectric effect, a photon impinging on a target is absorbed and produces the emission of an electron if the photon energy is equal or higher than the electron binding energy. In X-ray diagnostics, an X-ray photon can transfer its energy to an electron of the innermost shell of the target (named K), producing its ejection. Then, an electron from an outer shell replaces the vacancy created in the K-shell, following the emission of an X-ray photon having energy equal to the energy difference between the two shells involved in the process. The electron binding energy associated to the K-shell is called K-edge. It assumes great importance since it is characteristic of the material and, at this energy, X-ray attenuation shows a discontinuous trend due to the increased probability of photoelectric effect.

In X-ray diagnostics, it is easy to discriminate between tissues with highly different densities, such as bones and fat. On the other hand, the naturally occurring X-ray attenuation is not sufficient to produce appreciable contrast differentiation between diseased districts and healthy tissue, such as in case of tumors. Contrast agents are generally required in order to generate images with the highest contrast to the surrounding tissue and can: i) increase CT sensitivity and enhance differentiation among different tissues, ii) provide specific biochemical information of a tissue, or iii) enable evaluation of tissue/organ function or performance.

Hence, specific contrast agents comprising high atomic number materials with proper K-edge are needed to employ this imaging technique in cancer diagnostic. The most commonly used contrast agents for CT are both ionic and non-ionic forms of iodine-based compounds. These compounds are systemically injected, quickly distributed in the body, and finally excreted un-metabolized through hepatobiliary/renal pathways.

These traditional contrast agents show several limitations, among which: i) induced adverse effects as kidneys and thyroids dysfunctions, ii) allergic reactions, and iii) diagnostic limitations due to body clearance, which sometimes is too fast for prolonged imaging applications [3, 4]. On this regard, nanoparticle formulations of standard contrast agents have been proposed to increase blood residence and provide passive targeting accumulations in solid tumors. Among these, named blood pools, iodine-loaded liposomes have demonstrated prolonged blood circulation with

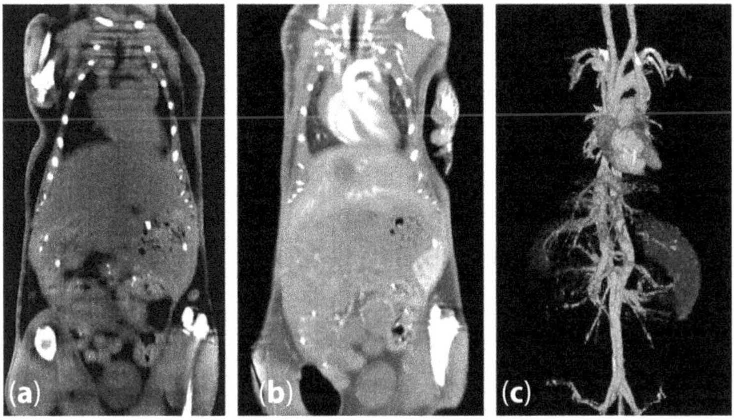

Figure 3.2 Micro CT images of mice before (a) and 6h after the injection of PEGylated Au NPs as contrast agents (b). Image (c) is the 3D volume rendered image [10].

respect to bare contrast media, providing high resolution images of mammary tumors *in vivo* in the rat model [5].

However, some drawbacks of iodinate agents are still retained even as nanosized formulation. In particular, the K-edge at 33 keV is highly unfavorable in many CT clinical exams, in which energies above 100 kVp are reached. Moreover, an effective diagnostic dose of iodinated contrast agent is usually in the molar concentration range. For example, an adult patient undergoing a selective coronary arteriography is injected intravenously with ~45 mL of Hexabrix (Mallinckrodt Imaging), a common clinically approved iodinated CT imaging agent solution, containing 24 g of ioxaglate (an equivalent to 14.4 g of iodine). To overcome these issues, alternative contrast agents based on inorganic NPs were investigated [6–9]. In particular, as shown in Figure 3.2, gold nanoparticles are an ideal radiopaque contrast media since gold has a high density, a high atomic number, and possess favorable K-edge at 80.7 keV [10]. For example, gold provides about 2.7 times greater contrast per unit weight than iodine. Furthermore, gold is inert, biocompatible, and is a straightforward material for the development of all-in-one nanoplatforms.

For example, Cole *et al.* reported *ex vivo* contrast-enhanced X-ray detection of breast microcalcifications through active targeting of hydroxyapatite employing bisphosphonate-modified gold NPs [11]. Zhang *et al.* achieved specific targeting of damaged bones with glutamic acid functionalized gold NPs, which accumulated in micro-cracks and resulting in a potential site-specific contrast agents for X-rays [12].

Direct comparison between commercial iodine-based contrast agents and gold NPs have been reported by many groups [13–15]. In particular, *Sun et al.* performed *in vivo* CT imaging of tumor bearing mice, observing a fivefold increase in the X-ray attenuation from the tumor 24h after tail injection of the NPs [16].

Interestingly, Dou *et al.* systematically investigated the relation between size of gold NPs in the range 3–50 nm and the CT contrast enhancement [17]. They observed that the attenuation didn't increase linearly with NPs size. Indeed, 13 nm NPs showed X-ray attenuation comparable with the attenuation produced by particles bigger than 40 nm. The findings were also confirmed by Monte Carlo simulations. The authors speculated that this behavior is related to the distribution of gold atoms in the particles, which is responsible for secondary interactions, *i.e.* attenuation of characteristic X-rays produced by primary X-ray-induced photoelectric effect. This idea was confirmed by investigations on gold atoms distribution in NPs by varying the NPs size.

It's worth mentioning that graphene oxide (GO) NPs have been very recently reported to serve as CT contrast agent when decorated by silver NPs. GO/Ag NPs provided 24h blood circulation time and afforded the *in vivo* contrast-enhanced CT imaging of lung, liver and kidneys. Notably, at the lowest dose (0.5 mg/kg of body weight), those nanoplatforms showed high specificity and sensitivity for the diagnosis of kidney dysfunctions, even 36 h after the injection [18].

3.1.2 Photoacoustic Imaging

Photoacoustic effect, discovered by Bell in 1880, is the generation of acoustic waves produced by thermal expansion of a piece of material, following absorption of photons. Briefly, when a medium is irradiated by a short-pulsed laser, part of the photon energy is dissipated as heat and temperature is increased locally, producing a raise of pressure. After cooling, pressure returns to its original value and this pressure waves, or sound waves, are detected by an ultrasound transducer.

Compared to ultrasonography, which is a sound in – sound out technique, Photoacoustic Imaging (PAI) is light in – sound out. PAI can be exploited by naturally occurring optical absorbers in the human tissues as endogenous contrast agents, such as hemoglobin and melanin. Several investigations on breast cancer patients are highlighted the great potential of PAI as clinical diagnostic tool (Figure 3.3) [19].

Commercially available low quantum yield dyes, such as methylene blue, indocyanine green and porphyrins, have been widely used as exogenous contrast media for PAI, since, upon light excitation, they produced enhanced local heating due to

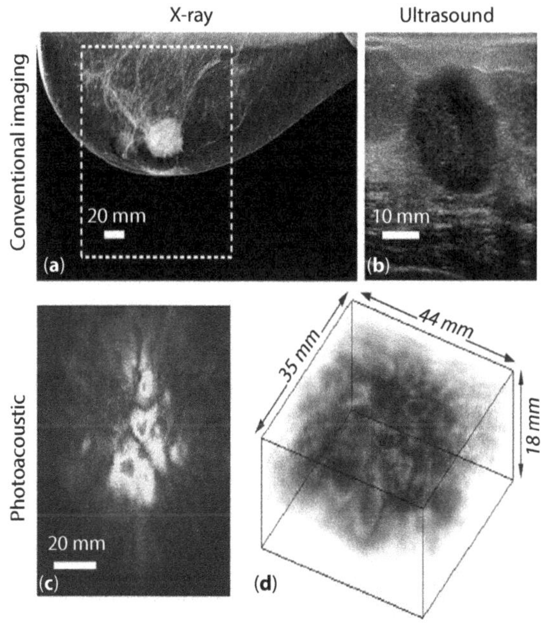

Figure 3.3 X-ray mammogram (a) of 69 year old woman infiltrating ductal carcinoma compared with ultrasonography scan image (b) and photoacoustic image (c) and 3D volume rendering (d) of the selected ROI [19]. Reprinted with permission from [19].

non-radiative decays. However, organic dyes have often low chemical stability, suffer from photo-bleaching, and are rapidly cleared from the body, being not suitable for prolonged PAI analyses. On this regard, nanomaterials, and in particular plasmonic metal NPs, have marked a major turning point in PAI technology, providing increased photostability, higher spatial resolution and selectivity.

Noble metal nanoparticles with anisotropic morphologies (nanoshells, nanocages, nanorods and branched NPs) are generally introduced as PAI contrast agents, due to their LSPRs in the NIR windows, allowing for deeper light penetration. In this regard, gold nanorods are ideal light-to-heat transducer. Indeed, they are among the most widely investigated nanomaterials for photoacoustic, mainly because of their tunable LSPRs in the NIR region and high extinction coefficient, which is almost all given by absorption. For example, Peng *et al.* have recently reported an *in vivo* PA investigation of both subcutaneous tumor and leg ischemia in mouse models by employing silica coated gold nanorods (Figure 3.4) [20].

Also, semiconducting nanoparticles, despite the absence of LSPRs, have demonstrated interesting behaviors as PAI probes. In particular, copper sulfide NPs have been employed as *in vivo* photoacoustic probes of brain, due to their strong absorption in the NIR region. Furthermore, copper sulfide NPs have allowed for *ex vivo* tissue imaging to up to 5 cm [21].

Organic nanomaterials have also been demonstrated to be suitable for PAI. For example, organic semiconducting polymeric NPs and dye functionalized carbon nanotubes have been reported to be excellent photoacoustic probes for *in vivo* cancer detection, exploiting their broad non-plasmonic absorption of visible to NIR light [22–24].

Agglomerates of self-organized small-molecules dyes, termed J-aggregates, were also shown to hold a good potential as PA probes with respect to single dyes, due to aggregation-induced self quenching and bathochromic shift [25, 26]. However, not

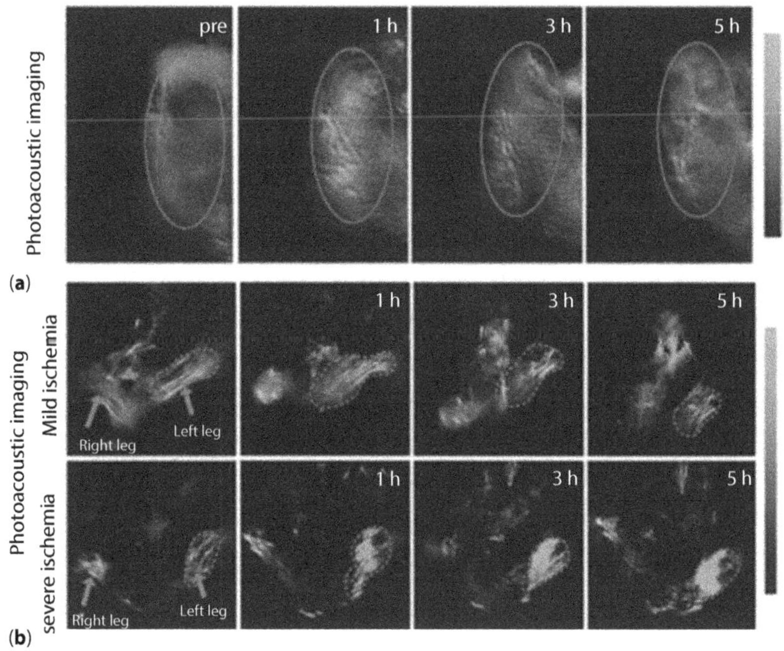

Figure 3.4 Photoacoustic imaging *in vivo* of mouse tumor (a) and ischemia (b) enhanced by silica coated gold nanorods [20]. Reproduced from [20] with permission of The Royal Society of Chemistry.

so many paper have been reported on the *in vivo* use of those aggregates, due to their poor stability into complex biological media [27–29]. Improvements in conformational stability of dye aggregates was recently achieved by embedding them into lipid vesicles. Moreover, their employment in *ex vivo* PAI of head and neck cancer was reported [28].

Of particular interest, a novel paradigm for the production of exogenous photoacoustic contrast media has been recently proposed by Avigo *et al.* [30]. The Authors have reported the *ex vivo* PAI detection of hybrid nano-architectures composed by plasmonic gold nanoparticles and organic dyes. The nano-architectures were designed to exploit the fluorescence quenching effect of gold NPs to increase the non-radiative decay of dyes, increasing the photoacoustic signals and avoiding the NPs re-shaping induced by irradiation.

3.1.3 Positron Emission Tomography

Positron Emission Tomography (PET) is a molecular imaging technique in which the final image is produced by the detection of photons arising from the annihilation of a positron with an electron in the tissue.

When a beta plus (positron) emitter radiotracer is injected in the patient, it spreads in the body and, following radioactive decay, it emits a positron with a certain kinetic energy. The positron loses energy mainly by Coulomb scattering, and when it reaches thermal equilibrium, it annihilates with a tissue electron, emitting two high energy photons (511 KeV) back-to-back. These photons are detected in coincidence by two oppositely located detectors and the annihilation point is calculated by reconstruction algorithms with a spatial resolution of 1–4 mm [31].

The calculated image is the map of radiotracer activity in the body, which is indicative of physiological and/or pathological activities of the patient. On this regard, the turning point in the employment of PET was due to the synthesis of the radiopharmaceutical fluorodeoxyglucose (^{18}F-FDG) [32]. ^{18}F-FDG is a glucose analog, whose uptake is directly correlated to organs metabolic activity.

^{18}F-FDG and many other glucose analogs have been also widely exploited in oncology for the diagnosis of a number of solid tumors. Indeed, many neoplasms are characterized by higher glucose consumption with respect to healthy tissues. However, PET contrast agents suffer from tissue non-specificity, poor accumulation and short blood circulation time, albeit several radiotracers based on physiological radioisotopes, such as ^{11}C, ^{13}N, ^{15}O and non-physiological ones like ^{64}Cu or ^{68}Ga have been synthesized. Moreover, spatial resolution is one of the most limiting features of this diagnostic tool, in particular on *in vivo* investigations.

These hurdles have been partially addressed with the rising of nano-radiopharmaceuticals, *i.e.* nanomaterials conjugated to radioisotopes which afforded the opportunity of: i) synergistic action between various imaging modalities, and ii) decoration by active targeting moieties.

Most of the radiolabeled nanomaterials employ chelating agents such as 1,4,7,10-tetraazacyclododecane-1,4,7,10-tetraacetic acid (DOTA), diethylenetriaminepentaacetic acid (DTPA), ethylenediaminetetraacetic acid (EDTA) or porphyrins, to load radioactive isotopes of metals, among which Cu, Y, Zr, In or Ga [34–36].

One of the most extensively used radioisotope, ^{64}Cu, has been conjugated both to organic NPs, as lipid vesicles and porphysomes, and to inorganic nanomaterials, such as gold NPs or silica NPs [37–42].

Unluckily, radiolabeling of nanomaterials by means of chelating agents has shown several drawbacks. In particular, the inherent instability of certain metal-chelator conjugates can result in losing the radioisotopes and subsequent non-specific binding to proteins [43]. Hence, an good knowledge in coordination chemistry is needed, in order to properly choose the most stable chelator for each radioisotope [34, 43].

Recently, new chelator-free strategies for radiolabeling of nanomaterials were developed. Several approaches for the production of intrinsically radiolabeled NPs have been summarized by Goel *et al.* They have identified four main synthetic strategies, among which an interesting post-synthetic labeling by proton beam induced nuclear reaction in metal oxides NPs [44]. Sun *et al.* reported a chelator-free radiolabeling route with ^{64}Cu on PEG stabilized gold NPs by directly reducing ^{64}Cu on gold NPs surface. They have also tested their feasibility as PET radiotracers *in vivo* [39]. Interestingly, Shi *et al.* have recently reported radiolabeling of nanographene by direct interaction between ^{64}Cu and π electrons following simple mixing of the two species in a proper buffer. This nanoplatform have demonstrated a good stability *in vitro*, in mouse serum, and was successfully employed in PET imaging in tumor-bearing mice [45].

Notably, a generalized route for post-radiolabeling ultrasmall iron oxide NPs was achieved by Boros *et al.*, who reported a heat-induced chelate-free labeling with ^{89}Zr, ^{64}Cu and ^{111}In. They have also reported an *in vivo* investigation on NPs biodistribution by combined CT/PET imaging on mouse models [46].

3.1.4 Magnetic Resonance Imaging

Magnetic Resonance Imaging (MRI) is a diagnostic technique based on the physical principle of Nuclear Magnetic Resonance (NMR), discovered by Bloch and Purcell in 1946, and for which they were awarded the Nobel prize in physics.

In this section we will briefly describe the principles that regulates the MRI, without getting into the physical details of the NMR, which are comprehensively discussed elsewhere [47, 48].

When a static magnetic field $\mathbf{B_0}$ is applied to a water-containing medium, the randomly oriented magnetic moments $\boldsymbol{\mu} = \gamma \mathbf{J}$ (where γ is the gyromagnetic ratio and $\mathbf{J}$ is the total angular momentum) of hydrogen nuclei, align along two anti parallel directions, being $J = \pm\hbar/2$, corresponding to two states[1] having energies $E = -\mu B_0$. $\mathbf{B_0}$ exerts a torque on $\boldsymbol{\mu}$, causing a precession of J about B_0 axis with an angular frequency $\omega_0 = \gamma B_0$ called Larmor frequency.

At the basis of the MRI, there are two main points: (i) Larmor frequency is peculiar for each element or isotope, and (ii) it is possible to collect the signal of a specific element or isotope by exciting the system with a radio frequency (RF) magnetic field orthogonal to $\mathbf{B_0}$, that matches its Larmor frequency. RF pulses

[1] Boltzmann statistic gives an estimate of the distribution of the high energy (N+) and low Energy (N−) states, at a given temperature T and at a given energy difference between the two states (ΔU):

$$\frac{N^+}{N^-} = e^{\left(-\frac{\Delta U}{KT}\right)}$$

where K is the Boltzmann constant.

cause the magnetic moments to flip from the low energy state, by an angle which depends on the pulse duration, revealing the magnetization of the system. When the RF pulse ends, the magnetization relax to its initial value, by producing itself an oscillating magnetic field, that is detected by a coil as a voltage signal, and is displayed as free-induction decay (FID).

The intrinsic time needed from the magnetization to return to its initial orientation after the end of the RF pulse is tissue-dependent, hence it is the source of contrast in MRI. In particular, two characteristic times are defined: (i) the transverse relaxation time, named T_2, and (ii) the longitudinal relaxation time, or T_1 (Figure 3.5).

T_1 is the time needed for the longitudinal component of magnetization to return to about 63% of its maximum value, *i.e.* spins lose energy by heat transfer to the environment,

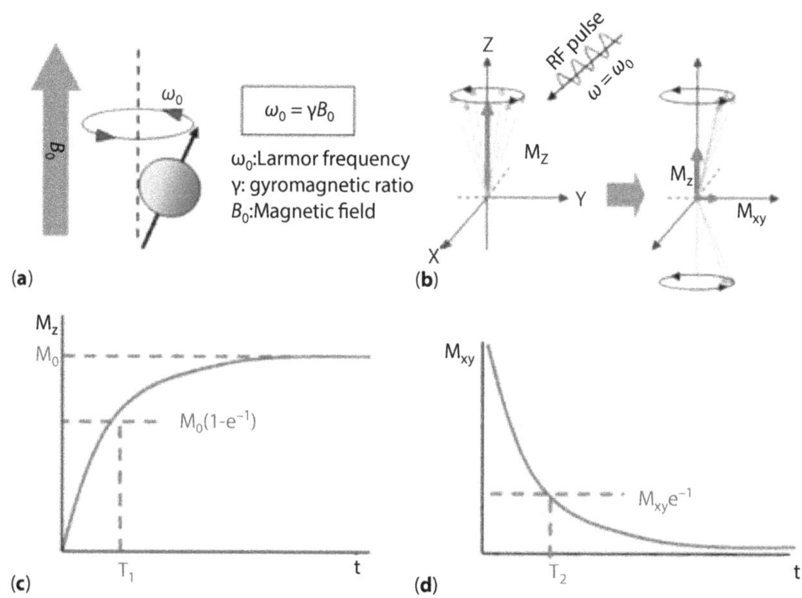

Figure 3.5 Nuclear spin precession about external static magnetic field axis (a), magnetization flip after the application of an RF pulse (b) and longitudinal and transversal magnetization relaxation law (c) and (d), respectively [49]. Reproduced from [49] with permission of John Wiley & Sons Inc.

favoring the low energy orientations. In biological tissues, T_1 ranges from tenths of second to few seconds, a relatively long time, because the energy transfer requires stimulation by surrounding molecules which produces a field oscillating at a frequency close to the Larmor's one.

T_2 is the time needed for the magnetization to decay to 37% of the value it possessed before the RF pulse, mainly through dephasing of ensembles of nuclear spins due to local magnetic field inhomogeneity.

The longitudinal and transverse relaxation times of protons in human tissues in both physiological and pathological states have been extensively investigated also as a function of temperature and magnetic field strength. From the tabulated reported by In 1986, Bottomley and co-workers have demonstrated that T_1 and T_2 values collected in neoplasms are usually quite increased respect to healthy tissues [50]. On the other hand, despite the increased water content of cancerous tissues, the differences of relaxation times due to necrosis, inflammations, or edemas respect to healthy tissues is negligible [51–54].

Hence, also for this imaging technique, contrast agents are needed to improve its efficiency for the detection of neoplasms.

The first nanoparticulate example of T_2 contrast agent was reported in 1986, when magnetite NPs at a concentration of 10 mg/kg body wt were injected intravenously in a dog model, inducing a net decrease in MRI contrast of liver and spleen [55]. Since nanosized iron oxide is superparamagnetic, it exhibits strong magnetization in presence of an external magnetic field, which disappears after the field is turned off. This magnetization creates local inhomogeneity of the magnetic fields, accelerating the nuclear spin coherence losing, thus shortening T_2. These tools are named negative contrast agent, because relaxation shortening produces a decrease in the signal intensity. Superparamagnetic Iron Oxide NPs (IONPs) are mainly exploited in detecting liver diseases, since IONPs are selectively internalized by Kupffer cells which are less numerous in tumor-bearing livers. Thus, after treatment with IONPs, damaged tissues appear brighter, *i.e.* with higher signal intensity, due to the poor uptake of negative contrast agents.

On this regard, Huang *et al.* investigated the T2 contrast enhancement *in vivo* depending on the IONPs size. They have performed MRI investigations with IONPs ranging from 8 to 65 nm on normal liver and hepatic lesions [56]. They found that 37 nm PVP-coated IONPs (HD: 100 nm) have the greatest contrast enhancement, in line with the maximum cellular uptake obtained with those NPs by macrophage cells (Figure 3.6).

Notably, Zhao *et al.* achieved effective T2 contrast enhancement and *in vivo* small liver tumors detection by employing anisotropic octapod IONPs. They reported stronger transverse relaxation of the octapods, in comparison with spherical IONPs of similar size, due to the strong magnetic field inhomogeneity induced by the anisotropic NPs under an external magnetic field, yielding stronger proton spin dephasing [57].

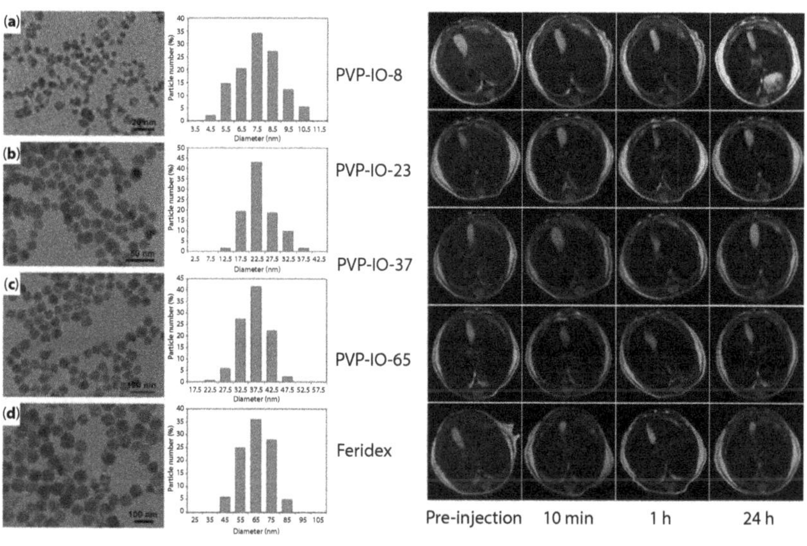

Figure 3.6 (Left) TEM images and size histograms of PVP-coated iron oxide NPs of sizes ranging from 7.6 to 65.3 nm and (Right) *in vivo* mouse liver MRI at different time steps after intravenous administration of the IONPs and the commercial contrast agent Feridex [56]. Reprinted with permission from [56]. Copyright 2010 American Chemical Society

Many other groups have dedicated a lot of efforts to the investigation of IONPs as T2 negative contrast agents for diagnosis of breast cancer, brain glioma, transplanted stem cells tracking and, very recently, lung cancer [58–61].

The contrast agents which shorten the T_1, *i.e.* increase the MRI signal, are named positive contrast agents. Most of them are based on nanoparticles comprising chelating agents for Gd(III). Indeed, Gd ions cannot be directly administered in organisms because of the high toxicity due to strong interference with calcium ions channels.

Advances in the use of Gd-based positive contrast agents were related to the introduction of gadolinium oxide (Gd_2O_3) NPs, gadolinium fluoride (GdF_3) and Gd-Si oxide NPs, which were reported to offer a higher longitudinal proton relaxivity and, at the same time, an improved safety profile with respect to Gd(III) chelates [62–64]. Park *et al.* reported the *in vivo* MRI of brain tumor in mice model by employing ultrasmall Gd_2O_3 NPs coated by D-glucuronic acid [65]. These NPs have demonstrated an increased relaxivity and a significant reduction of toxicity respect to Gd(III) chelates.

Notably, Li *et al.* have recently reported the production of dual modal MRI contrast agents for both T_1 and T_2, by synthesizing Fe_3O_4/Gd_2O_3 core/shell nanocubes. Although other groups had previously reported the synthesis of dual modal MRI contrast agents, this was the first report of cubically-shaped NPs containing both iron and gadolinium [66–68]. Holding relaxivities about two folds higher than Fe_3O_4 nanocubes and Gd_2O_3 NPs, these hybrid nanostructures were exploited for MRI in murine models, showing high positive and negative contrast enhancement in the liver and producing negligible cytotoxicity and no induced morphological changes in both normal and tumor cell lines [69].

3.1.5 Raman-Based Diagnostics

Raman spectroscopy is an analytical technique that allows for fingerprint identification of chemical species constituting complex biological samples. Moreover, cells or tissues that are subjected to biochemical alterations due to diseases can be distinguished from healthy tissue by significant changes in the Raman spectra. Raman spectroscopy can provide fingerprints of tissues at molecular level, increasing the interest among scientists for its potential as promising diagnostic tool.

Raman spectroscopy relies on the collection of electromagnetic radiation triggered by a laser that is scattered either elastically or inelastically upon interaction with a material. The scattered light is collected and its intensity is plotted against: i) the frequency shift (Raman shift) with respect to incident light, or ii) the inverse of wavelength, named wave number, which is usually expressed in cm^{-1} (Figure 3.7).

Most of the light is scattered elastically (Rayleigh scattering), whereas a photon every 10^6 to 10^8 exchanges energy with the medium through phonons mediated scattering processes [70]. These inelastically scattered photons give rise to the Stokes and anti-Stokes peaks in the Raman spectra, corresponding to light which have released energy to the analyte, or acquired energy from it, respectively.

Raman spectroscopy reveal the vibrational structure of the sample, since after having interacted inelastically with photons, the molecules are in a vibrational state which is different from the initial one, and the Raman shifts match exactly the energy difference between initial and final vibrational level of the analyte.

Raman peaks are narrow and can be associated to specific vibrations of chemical bonds [71]. Thus, Raman spectra depict a detailed chemical fingerprint of the molecular system under investigation, allowing for its rapid identification and providing sensitivity to conformational changes. Nevertheless, the detection of chemicals in complex biological media is limited by several drawbacks, such as the inherent low sensitivity of Raman technique towards electronically saturated systems, *i.e.* carbohydrates lipids or amino acids [72]. Indeed, Raman selection rules expects that the higher the polarizability of the analyte, the more intense are the Raman peaks, meaning that the

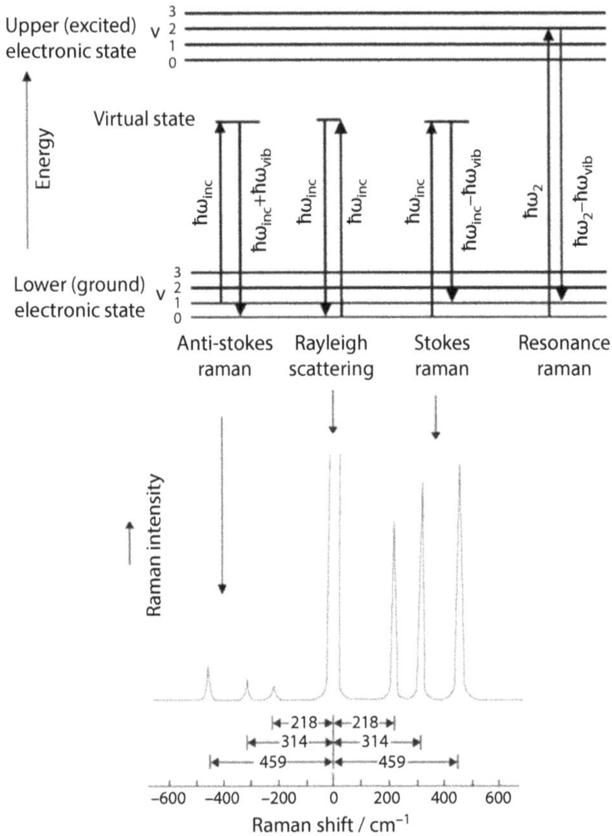

Figure 3.7 Jablonski diagram showing vibrational energy levels involved in Raman scattering (top) and Raman spectrum of CCl_4 (bottom) [73]. Reprinted with permission from [73]. Copyright 2016 Springer Nature.

best detectable species are molecules with extended π-electron systems, such as aromatic moieties.

A huge step forward towards increasing the sensitivity and selectivity of Raman spectroscopy was made after the experimental evidence that Raman spectra acquired with an excitation source whose frequency is closely matched an electronic transition of the analyte showed enhanced peak intensities [74]. This phenomenon, named resonance Raman effect, was exploited by anchoring chromophores to sites of interests, to achieve signal enhancement and high selectivity towards specific vibrational modes.

However, labeling biological samples of interests with small dyes to exploit the resonance enhancement have shown some drawbacks that prevented Raman spectroscopy to be employed as effective diagnostic tool. For example, the fluorescence background significantly reduces Raman signals collection. Indeed, typical fluorescence cross section of chromophores are in the range 10^{-17}–10^{-16}, while the respectively Raman cross sections are usually in the range 10^{-30}–10^{-25} cm^2 [75]. This issue is of particular importance in resonance Raman, since the laser source is energetically close to the electronic transition, increasing the probability of fluorescent emission, whose intensity and spectral broadening can easily overwhelm Raman peaks [76]. Moreover, the introduction of exogenous tags can potentially interfere with physiological conditions.

On this regard, metal nanoparticles have represented the turning point in the development of Raman-based highly sensitive diagnostics due to: i) the fluorescence quenching properties of some metals, and ii) the Raman signals enhancement [77–79].

Surface Enhanced Raman Scattering (SERS) pushed the inherently insensitive Raman spectroscopy to unprecedented levels of sensitivity thanks to the giant signal enhancement, up to 10^{15}, that allow to single molecule detection [80]. The physical mechanisms at the basis of SERS are today well understood and arise both from the local electromagnetic field enhancement owing to the plasmonic effect (physical enhancement), and from an electronic coupling between the analyte and metal surface (chemical enhancement). The enhancement factors are strongly dependent on the SERS substrates, analytes and excitation wavelength; however, this subject is beyond the scope of this book, and it is comprehensively reviewed elsewhere [81].

Colloidal gold and silver NPs are among the most investigated SERS-active substrates for non-invasive early diagnosis of diseases, and many groups reported their use for the detection of clinically relevant analytes from biological fluids, such as cancer related proteins and DNA biomarkers [82–87].

The development of noble metal NPs whose plasmonic response is shifted up to near infrared, and the synthesis of novel NIR Raman-active molecules have allowed for the translation of SERS based diagnostics *in vivo*, owing to the greater penetration depth in tissues of NIR laser sources [88, 89]. Zhang *et al.* reported the *in vivo* SERS detection of tumors in a mouse model, by employing dye-labeled silica/polymer coated gold nanorods. Imaging was performed by mapping the intensity of one SERS peak (508 cm^{-1}) of 3,3'-diethylthiatricarbocyanine iodide (DTTC) which revealed an increased intensity at tumor sites due to accumulation of nanorods [90]. DTTC dye was also exploited as Raman reporter by many other groups [91, 92]. For instance, Conde *et al.* reported *in vivo* tumor inhibition and spectroscopic contour detection, *i.e.* theranostics, with a nanosystem composed by 90 nm gold NPs capped with DTTC as Raman reporter and an antibody-drug conjugate in mouse bearing xenograft tumors [93].

Tian *et al.* achieved *in vivo* real time SERS tracking of Mitoxantrone (MTX) chemotherapeutic drug release in a lung cancer mouse model, by employing NIR resonant gold nanostars as SERS probes. Notably, dye-labeling of gold nanostars was not needed, since drug release was imaged by evaluating the SERS intensity of aromatic C-C stretching of the MTX itself, which acted both as therapeutic and imaging tool [94].

Interestingly, Gandra *et al.* have recently synthesized gold/gold core/shell SERS nanoprobes with tunable interstitial gap that exhibited plasmon resonances at 785 nm, which showed exceptional stability in physiological conditions both *in vitro* and *in vivo* over 24 hours, allowing for prolonged non-invasive imaging of tumors in a mouse model (Figure 3.8) [95].

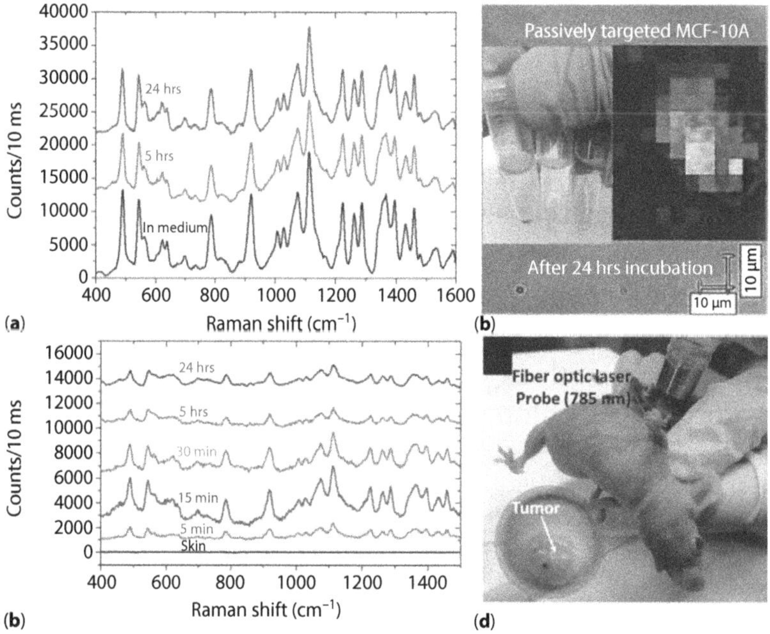

Figure 3.8 SERS spectra of gold based nanoprobes incubated with cultured breast epithelial cells during 24 h (a) and SERS mapping on a single cell (b). SERS spectra of nanoprobes over time *in vivo* after intratumoral injection (c). Experimental setup for *in vivo* SERS (d) [95]. Reproduced from [95] with permission of The Royal Society of Chemistry

3.2 Therapy

3.2.1 Chemotherapy

Chemotherapy, literally a therapy based on chemicals, is referred to the administration of cytotoxic chemical agents for the treatment of neoplasms. The first reported use of chemotherapeutic drugs for healing cancer dates back to 1940s, when nitrogen mustards were employed for the treatment of a patient lymphoma [96].

Chemotherapy is often used as adjuvant therapy after a surgical treatment, or as preoperative therapy with the aim of reducing the tumor volume before the surgery. In advanced stages, chemotherapy is used only as palliative care for providing relief from painful symptoms and slightly increase patients' life expectancy [97].

The majority of drugs employed in chemotherapy interact with cells functions, altering their growth and division. A huge class of chemotherapeutic drugs, belonging from nitrogen mustard, is alkylating agents, which are chemicals that add an alkyl group to important biological macromolecules, including DNA, inhibiting their normal functions and causing double strand breaks, which eventually lead to cell death.

Another chemotherapeutic drug that inhibits DNA functions is cis-diamminedichloroplatinum (II) (cisplatin). It acts as DNA crosslinker, mainly causing intrastrand cross-link. Cisplatin attaches to DNA purine bases, preventing the opening of DNA double helices. Cisplatin was introduced in clinical investigations in 1971 and dominated the therapy of ovarian and testicular cancers for decades [98]. Many cisplatin analogues have been synthesized during the years, even though only cis diammine (1,1-cyclobutanecarboxylate) platinum (II), known as carboplatin, have received clinical approval owing to its reduced side effects and enhanced chemotherapeutic activity [99].

Another important class of chemotherapeutic drugs comprises antimetabolites, which include: i) cytarabine, employed for the treatment of acute myeloid leukemia, and ii) gemcitabine, a prodrug which is converted to its active form inside the cells upon kinase phosphorylation [100, 101]. These chemotherapeutics inhibit the nucleic acids synthesis. Antimetabolites include either: i) analogues of pyrimidines and purines, which replace the naturally occurring bases that constitute the building blocks in the synthesis of DNA and RNA impairing their production, or ii) antifolates, which are antagonists of folic acid, an essential vitamin in the production and repair of nucleic acids.

Topoisomerase inhibitors are a class of chemotherapeutic drugs that includes doxorubicin (DOX). DOX is a natural antibiotic extracted from soil fungi, whose cytotoxicity is produced by several mechanisms including: i) DNA intercalation, which inhibits the progression of the enzyme topoisomerase II, and ii) generation of cytotoxic free radicals, such as peroxides and superoxides [102].

Chemotherapeutics can induce cells death also by destabilizing microtubule polymerization, leading to their anomalous production or deficiency. Since microtubules play a pivotal role in a number of cellular activities, including proliferation, adhesion, migration and intracellular transport, an anomalous polymerization heavily influences the cell cycle, inducing apoptosis. One of the most successful chemotherapeutic drug acting on microtubules is paclitaxel, whose anticancer activity relies in the stabilization of microtubules reducing their dynamism and causing the block of mitotic phase by leading to apoptotic death [103].

Unluckily, none of these drugs is tumor-specific. Thus, upon administration, they spread all over the body causing severe adverse effects, in particular to fast proliferating cells: blood cells in the bone marrow, hair follicles, reproductive systems and tissues belonging to the digestive apparatus.

Hence, common side effects include hair loss, asthenia, headache, nausea and vomiting, severe blood disorders such as thrombocytopenia and leucopenia, diffused pain, cognitive dysfunctions including memory and attention loss or nerve damages. Moreover, some adverse effects may last for months/year after chemotherapy treatment, seriously prejudicing patient's life quality and expectancy [104].

Overall, chemotherapeutic treatment is often doomed to failure due to the occurrence of drug resistance, either because of: i) inefficient drug distribution in tumor tissues, or ii) through molecular efflux pumps which provide extrusion of the drugs from the cells [105].

Therefore, increasing efforts are devoted to achieve localized and enhanced anticancer activity of drugs. Nanotechnology offer a concrete possibility for the development of targeted chemotherapeutics, owing to: i) passive accumulation of nanomaterials at tumor site through Enhanced Permeability and

Retention effect (EPR, see chapter 2), and ii) combination of multiple drugs on the same nanoplatform.

During the last decades, a plethora of works were published on this subject, establishing nanomedicine as one of the most exciting field of academic research.

After the successful encapsulation of drugs in liposomes in 1973, one of the first significant clinical trials of chemotherapeutics nanoformulation was reported in 1996 by Nortfelth and co-workers [106, 107]. They proposed a liposome comprising doxorubicin against Kaposi's sarcoma and reported an accumulation of liposome-encapsulated doxorubicin in the target to up to 11.4 times more respect to standard doxorubicin.

Triggered by this results, several liposomal formulations comprising various drugs, among which cisplatin and paclitaxel, have been produced, and, notably, there are 16 liposomal drug formulations that are currently clinically approved, among which six are treatments for cancer-related diseases [108–110]. Also metal NPs, in particular gold nanostructures have been extensively employed as drug carriers owing to their biocompatibility, the straightforward surface functionalization, and the possible on-demand drug-release by exogenous or endogenous stimuli [111, 112]. Owing to the high affinity of gold surface towards thiols, endogenously triggered release can be *in situ* achieved due to the difference between intracellular (1–10 mM) and extracellular (1–5 μM) glutathione (GSH) concentration. Indeed, GSH can act either as a reducing agent, cleaving moieties linked through disulfide bonds to gold surface, or as substituting coating agent, replacing the original surface capping layer [113].

Stimuli responsive gold NPs have been also engineered to be triggered by external laser irradiation [114–116]. On this regard, effective spatio-temporal control over release of cargo molecules was achieved through 1,2,3 triazolic systems functionalized 30 nm gold NPs, which allowed for externally triggered payload release inside target cells through synergic action of irradiation with 561 nm laser and local electromagnetic field enhancement induced by LSPR stimulation [117].

Polymer nanomaterials are other interesting candidates for nanoparticle-mediated chemotherapy. The most promising are PLGA NPs, due to sustained release properties, low toxicity and high encapsulation capability of hydrophobic moieties [118–122]. Very recently, Rodgers and collaborators reported the synthesis and *in vivo* application of PLGA NPs comprising both paclitaxel and cisplatin. They found that co-delivery of the two encapsulated drugs enhanced the chemotherapeutic efficacy against lung tumors relatively to both free drugs combination and also combined administration of single drug loaded NPs [123].

Owing to biocompatibility, easy designing, high drug loading and biodegradation to nontoxic byproducts, silica NPs hold a prominent position in promising chemotherapeutic development [124]. During the last year many groups have reported chemotherapy applications of silica NPs both *in vitro* and *in vivo*, also exploiting strategies for selective drug release, either by endogenous or exogenous stimuli [125–130].

In this context, Zhang and co-workers have recently reported a strategy for synthesizing biodegradable silica nanocarriers for gene/drug co-delivery, whose release is related to GSH-induced biodegradation [131]. In particular, they have employed a modified Stöber method for the synthesis of their nanoplatforms. DOX was mixed to tetraethyl orthosilicate (TEOS) and disulfide bond-bridged silane (BTOCD) in presence of ammonia in order to obtain drug-loaded silica nanoparticles in one step, which exhibited accelerated degradation kinetics owing to the instable disulfide bridges in the silica matrix. Upon proper surface functionalization with targeting moieties, these smart nanoplatforms were successfully exploited for *in vivo* therapy on glioma tumor bearing mice, inducing an interesting decrease in tumor size after the treatment compared free DOX (Figure 3.9).

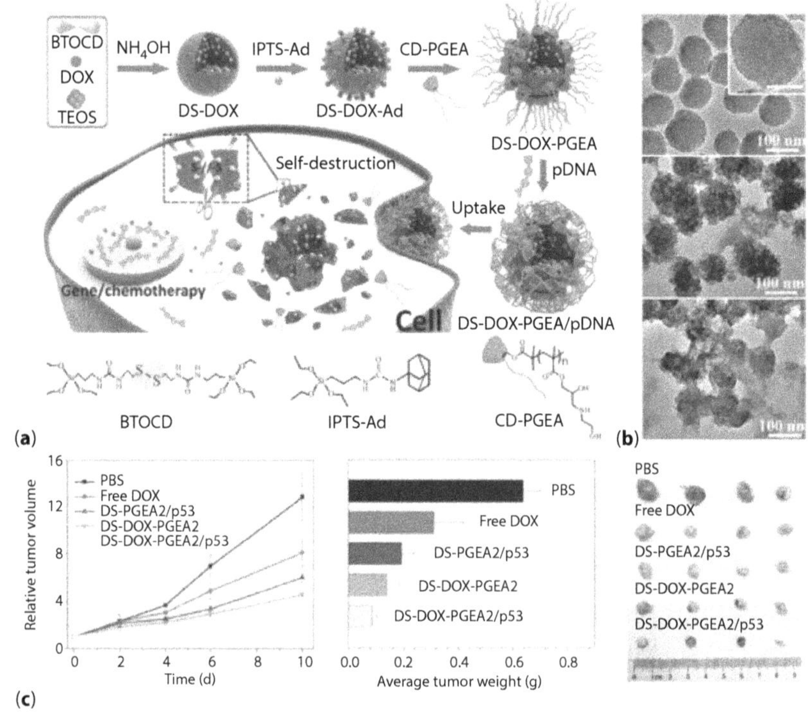

Figure 3.9 (a) Scheme of the synthesis and self-destruction mechanisms with subsequent drug release of doxorubicin (DOX)-loaded mesoporous silica NPs (DS) coated with CD-PGEA targeting agent (DS-DOX-PGEA). (b) TEM images of DS-DOX-PGEA in ethanol (top) and their degradation after 1 day (center) and 4 days (bottom) in a PBS solution of glutathione. (c) Tumor relative shrinking (left) and average weight (center) after 10 days of treatment with PBS (black), free doxorubicin (red), DS-PGEA coated with p53 gene for inhibiting tumor proliferation (blue), DS-DOX-PGEA (green) and DS-DOX-PGEA coated with p53 (yellow), and picture of the treated tumors *ex vivo* (right) [131]. Reproduced from [131] with permission of John Wiley & Sons Inc.

A remarkable result was very recently reported by Dai *et al.*. They synthesized silica coated rare earth up-converting NPs able to emit photons at shorter wavelength than the absorbed ones, producing multidrug release upon irradiation with near infrared light source [132]. In their work, DOX was loaded into porous silica shell. Pores were closed by a photoactivatable moiety linked to a cisplatin prodrug. After irradiation with 808 nm laser, the up-converting NPs emitted UV photons that triggered the conversion of cisplatin prodrug into its active form, while simultaneously opening the gates for doxorubicin release. These multiphoton activated double-drug delivery nanoplatforms were exploited for *in vivo* chemotherapy on tumor bearing Kunming mice, reporting significant tumor shrinking while not producing any scars on the skin at the irradiation site, due to the short duration of laser pulses which prevent overheating.

3.2.2 Hyperthermia

HyperThermia (HT) is an ancient therapeutic procedure consisting in raise the temperature of the diseased body areas, or the whole body, to improve its healing. It is typically combined to other therapeutic techniques. HT is commonly defined as temperature increase up to 45 °C, as higher temperature treatments fall into the thermal ablation techniques [133].

For the treatment of cancer-related diseases, HT is either supplied alone or in support to chemo- and radiation therapy, enhancing their therapeutic action. HT, indeed, was proven to enhance the cytotoxic effect of many chemotherapeutic drugs, including the most widely used cisplatin, Doxorubicin, Paclitaxel and Gemcitabine, although the mechanisms underlying these enhancements are still not fully understood [134–137].

Interestingly, HT does not bear significant effect on cultured cancer cells viability, while induce a significant effect *in vivo* due to the vasculature of solid tumors, the highly acidic environments of neoplasms, and the usual marked hypoxia that cancer cells suffer [138].

HT treatment of solid tumors is locally supplied by either external electromagnetic or ultrasound sources or by heating the target with a hot fluid. Whole body HT is performed typically to treat diffused metastatic cancers, for which a large area needs to be covered.

The effectiveness of HT treatment against tumors has been ascribed to several temperature-dependent biological mechanisms, including impaired DNA double strand break repair, misregulation of gene expression, increased mitochondrial reactive oxygen species (ROS) production, cytoskeleton disruption resulting in altered intracellular transport, antitumor immune response activation and many others [139–144].

Despite the benefits brought by HT in oncology, there are several issues to be addressed to enable its widespread use in clinics. Indeed, the localization of the treatment is difficulty reached and not all the body' districts are equally sensitive to temperature increase. For example, many tissues are unaffected by prolonged HT treatments (1 hour at 44 °C), while milder HT conditions (42 °C for 40 minutes) irreversibly damage the central nervous system [145]. Furthermore, heat exposure of large areas, up to whole body, results in thermo-tolerance development due to heat shock proteins (HSP) concentration increase, significantly reducing the benefits of repeated HT treatments [146].

Hence, also this technique needs an increased specificity of action to enhance the treatment effectiveness. One important step forward toward this goal was accomplished through the engineering of light-responsive NPs that produced heat upon interaction with non-ionizing radiation.

NPs assisted light-induced heat is mainly achieved by employing nanomaterials composed by low quantum yield dyes or plasmonic metal NPs or semiconductor quantum dots or carbon-based nanomaterials, each one relying on different physiochemical light-to-heat conversion mechanisms [147].

Gold nanorods (Figure 3.10) are among the most widely used nanomaterials for PT owing to: i) an exceptional conversion efficiency (namely the ratio between absorption and extinction cross sections), and ii) their finely tunable LSPR up to the NIR

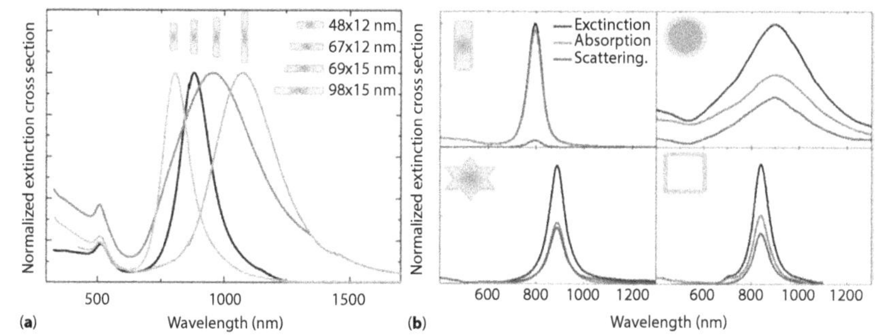

Figure 3.10 (a) Extinction cross section spectra of gold nanorods of different aspect ratio and (b) clockwise, comparison between simulated extinction, scattering and absorption cross sections of gold nanorods, nanoshells, nanocages and nanostars of representative sizes [147]. Reproduced from [147] with permission of The Royal Society of Chemistry

biological windows. One of the earliest example was published by Huang *et al.* in 2006 [148]. They reported a selective photothermal destruction of cultured cancer cells incubated with gold nanorods by irradiating at 800 nm in 40–200 mW power range, demonstrating an interesting dependence between nanomaterial uptake and cell apoptosis. A significant was achieved by Li *et al.*, who perform *in vitro* photothermal investigations on gold nanorods-incubated HeLa cells by employing a circular polarized pulsed femtosecond laser beam [149].

Remarkably, Choi *et al.* developed smart chitosan-conjugated pluronic acid-based nanocarriers containing aggregates of gold nanorods, which were reported to yield *in vivo* higher photothermal efficiency relatively to single nanorods, achieving an apparently complete tumor resorption on bilateral tumor bearing mice [150].

In the last decade, several other investigations on *in vivo* effectiveness of gold nanorods for PTT have been reported [151–154]. In particular, very recently, Zhao and co-workers produced dual-stimuli responsive and reversibly pH-triggered gold nanorods for tumor-selective PTT [155]. Nanorods were functionalized by a pH-switchable asymmetric cyanine dye, which provide additional PT effect and fluorescence imaging, and a metalloproteinases targeting peptide, achieving PTT in mice bearing subcutaneous tumors (Figure 3.11).

Other gold nanostructures employed for both *in vitro* and *in vivo* PTT include nanoshells, branched NPs, nanocages, nanocubes and the unusual gold/silica geometry named nanomatryoshkas [156–162]. The latter has shown higher PT transduction efficiency in a direct *in vivo* comparative study against gold nanoshells.

Furthermore, PTT was obtained also by employing other plasmonic metal nanomaterials (such as Pt, Pd and, very recently, titanium nitride NPs), carbon-based nanomaterials

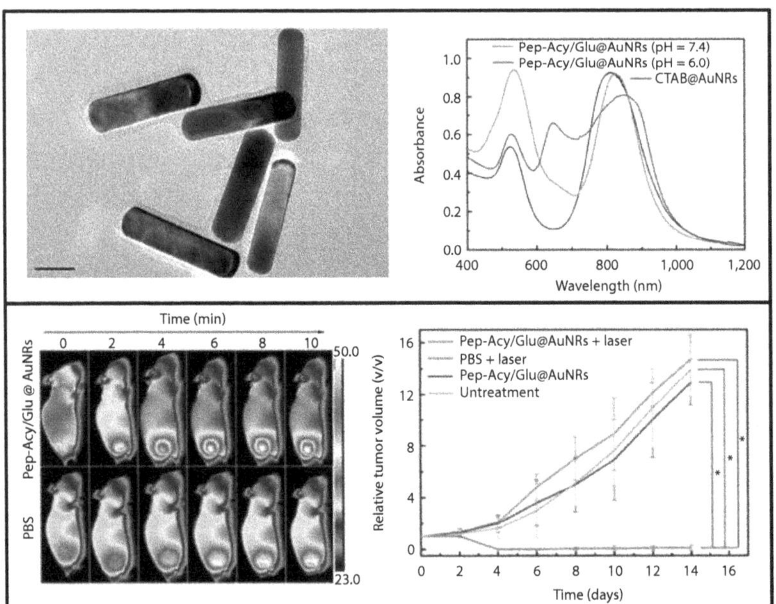

Figure 3.11 Upper panel: TEM image of cyanine/peptide/glucosamine-functionalized gold nanorods (Pep-Acy/Glu@AuNRs, left) and their absorbance spectra at neutral and acidic pH compared to absorbance of CTAB coated gold nanorods (right). Bottom panel: representative thermal images of mice treated with Pep-Agy/Glu@AuNRs or with PBS upon exposure to 808 nm laser irradiation (left) and relative tumor size variation for each group of mice (right) [155]. Reproduced from [155] with permission of John Wiley & Sons Inc.

(including carbon nanotubes, graphene and graphene oxide NPs), semiconductor and polymeric NPs [163–176].

Another class of external-triggered heat-generating nanomaterials is represented by magnetic NPs. Magnetic NPs can produce heat under the action of an alternating magnetic field. The heating efficiency is proportional to the frequency of the magnetic field. The physical principles at the basis of heat generation by magnetic nanomaterials are related to the NPs size and the strength of the applied magnetic field, and can be summarized into three mechanisms: (i) eddy currents, (iii) hysteresis loss and (iii) Neel and Brownian relaxation.

Eddy currents have usually a low contribute to magnetic NPs enhanced HT because the NPs small size and their low electrical conductivity [177, 178]. In turn, heat generation by hysteresis losses is ascribed merely to thermodynamic conservation of energy: when an external magnetization is raised from $\mathbf{M}_0$ to a certain value $\mathbf{M}_1$ by an external magnetic field $\mathbf{H}$, if the reversal of $\mathbf{H}$ does not bring the magnetization back to $\mathbf{M}_0$, *i.e.* in case of hysteresis, the nonzero difference of internal magnetic energy between initial and final state equals the work made by $\mathbf{H}$ plus heat. Hysteresis losses occur both in multi-domain materials, due to domain walls reorganization, and in single-domain ones, according to Stoner and Wohlfarth, when magnetic anisotropy is so high that coherent reversal of atomic magnetic moments is inhibited [179].

Heating by single-domain NPs occurs also through magnetic moment orientation fluctuations either due to Brownian physical motion of the NPs in the fluid or owing to fluctuations of the magnetic moment within the particles (Neel fluctuations). Upon application of an external alternating magnetic field, both the phenomena occur with different relaxation times, though efficient thermal transduction of magnetic energy is achieved only when Neel relaxation is not the dominant process [180].

The first report of magnetic NPs assisted HT goes back to 1957, when IONPs of size varying between 20 and 100 nm exposed to a radio frequency alternating magnetic field were shown to produce heat-induced necrosis in lymph nodes at the concentration of 5 mg NPs per gram of tissue [181]. Since then, the physical mechanisms at the basis of heat generation by magnetic NPs have been deeply investigated, with a particular focus on understanding collective effects produced by interparticle (*e.g.* dipolar) interactions, of undoubted relevance for practical cases [182–184]. Indeed, Dennis and co-workers provided the experimental evidences of the enhanced heat generation produced by collective interactions of magnetite NPs, which were successfully employed for *in vivo* HT, leading to almost complete regression of mammary tumor in mouse model [185].

Recent efforts in addressing the challenge of controlling interparticle interactions to achieve enhanced HT efficiency were published by Andreu *et al.*, who reported the synthesis of 1D worm-like and 2D spherical surface arrangements of magnetite NPs, employing silica and PLGA nanocarriers, respectively [186]. They have demonstrated that the geometrical arrangement is the key-feature for the thermal generation efficiency, rather than the concentration of magnetite NPs.

With the aim of combining more potential therapies in a single nanoplatform, synergistic action of PT and magnetic assisted HT was achieved by synthesizing NPs bearing both plasmonic and magnetic features. It was demonstrated that upon exposure of these hybrid magnetoplasmonic NPs to laser irradiation and radiofrequency magnetic field, the cumulative effect of bimodal PT and HT led to a remarkable local increase of temperature *in vivo*, reaching 48 °C at the tumor site in a mouse model (Figure 3.12) [187].

Ding *et al.* demonstrated the enhanced therapeutic effect produced by hybrid silver-IONPs upon HT treatment. They have observed that the presence of silver together with magnetic NPs, either in a core shell or dimeric arrangement, led to an

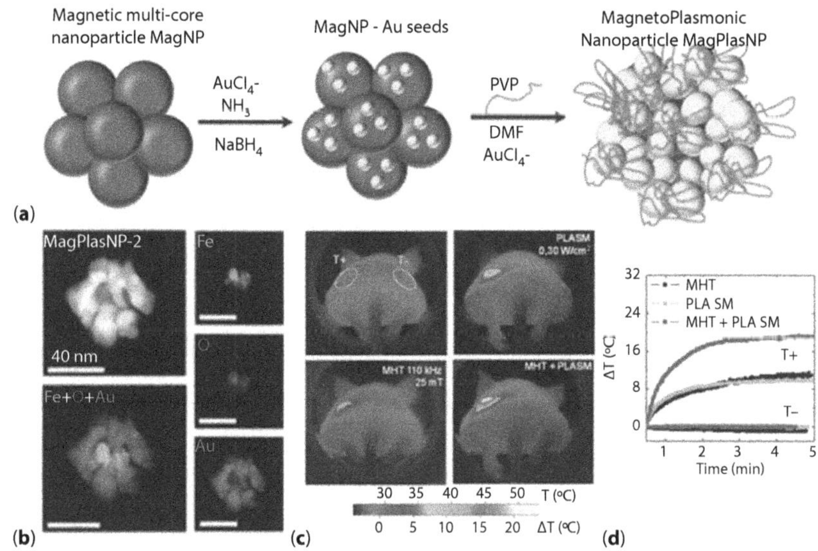

Figure 3.12 (a) Scheme of the synthesis of nanoplatforms bearing both plasmonic and magnetic features (MagPlasmNP), (b) HAADF image and EELS elemental analysis of MagPlasmNP and (c) temperature map of mouse model subjected to HT treatments upon intratumoral injection of MagPlasmNP due to laser stimulation (PLASM), RF magnetic field (MHT) or synergistic applications of the two (MHT+PLASM). (d) Plot of temperature variation at tumor site containing MagPlasmNP (T+) and at control tumor (T−) [187]. Reproduced from [187] with permission of The Royal Society of Chemistry.

increased tumor suppression, which the authors attributed to the synergistic effect of magnetic HT and silver ions release triggered by the increase in temperature [188]. Several groups have also reported the synthesis of complex nanoplatforms comprising both drugs and magnetic NPs, that have the potential for combined HT/chemotherapy or for HT-triggered drug release [189–192].

A plethora of other *in vivo* investigations on NPs assisted magnetic hyperthermia have been introduced during the last years, confirming the excitement of the scientific community towards this promising non-invasive treatment [193–196].

3.2.3 Radiotherapy

Along with chemotherapy, radiation therapy (or radiotherapy, RT) is one of the most employed cancer treatment. Indeed, about 60% of oncological patients experienced RT sessions, either as primary or adjuvant therapy. In RT, high doses of ionizing radiations (X-rays, γ-rays, hadrons) are administered either with external beams or with radiation sources injected in the body (brachytherapy), to shrink tumors.

The effect of RT is related to either directly damaging fundamental biological macromolecules, or by producing free radicals, such as reactive oxygen species (ROS). Even though ionizing radiations induce damage indiscriminately to healthy and diseased tissues, cancer cells are often unable to recover from DNA damage owing to inefficient repair pathways [197]. Hence, RT is administered in multiple sessions at low doses, repeated after a rest period which allows only healthy tissues to recover from the inflicted non-lethal damage.

Nonetheless, RT involving low radiation doses is often inefficient against cancer, since many tumors display an inherent resistance to ionizing radiations, owing to their hypoxic environment which severely limits ROS-induced cytotoxicity. On the other hand, an aggressive treatment plan could effectively damage tumors irreversibly while, in turn, increasing the likelihood of off-target injuries.

Hence, increase and localize the radiation dose at the tumor site by employing radiosensitizers is one of the most sparkling field of investigation. On this way, inorganic NPs of high atomic number elements are particularly suitable for this task, owing to their increased cross section for photoelectric effect [198].

Kobayashi *et al.* have reviewed the mechanisms at the basis of radiation dose enhancement by high-Z elements, stressing the role of Auger effect (a secondary low energy electron cascade emission that ensue photoionization) as the main responsible of local increase of dose deposition [199]. Also, although not explicitly referred to the Auger cascade, early experiments on increased radicals production in close proximity of 2 nm gold NPs irradiated by X-rays, have demonstrated the release of secondary electrons [200].

Gold NPs displayed interesting radiosensitization features even at radiation energies in the megavolt range, at which the photoelectric effect becomes negligible [201]. This feature has raised reasonable questions regarding the physical bases of radiosensitization of gold NPs, since it cannot be completely addressed to the high photon absorption cross section of gold nor to gold-induced oxidative stress [202]. Recently, it has been reported that the radiosensitization ability of gold NPs can be potentially influenced by their shape [203]. Indeed, it was observed on living cells experiments that gold nanospheres, nanorods and nanospikes of similar sizes produces different radiosensitization enhancements upon X-rays irradiation, with the highest enhancement reported for spherical gold NPs. Despite that, it is worth to notice that when the sensitization enhancement was normalized by the cellular uptake the differences become negligible, revealing that the increase in radiobiological effects is solely dependent by the increased NPs cellular internalization.

Notwithstanding incomplete knowledge of the radiosensitization mechanisms, gold NPs are a very promising and the most investigated nanomaterials for enhanced RT. Indeed, in the last years, plenty of works report both *in vitro* and *in vivo* investigations [204–210]. Nonetheless, other materials have been explored for enhanced RT, including cerium oxide, hafnium oxide, bismuth sulfide, gadolinium and silver [211–220]. In particular, Liu and co-workers investigated the radiosensitizing properties of silver NPs by a direct benchmark against gold NPs of the same size (15 nm), surface coating and concentration, upon irradiation by X-rays at megavolt energies [221]. Radiosensitizing efficacy of both

NPs was tested *in vivo* on glioma-bearing mice after intratumoral administration, finding that Ag NPs yielded significant increase in antiglioma activity when irradiated at 6 MV X-rays, compared to their Au counterparts. The authors suggest that this enhanced radiosensitization could be ascribed to the increased level of autophagy induced by silver NPs with respect to gold.

However, several studies on the cytotoxic effects induced by silver nanostructures indicate that the radiosensitization properties of Ag NPs are likely a consequence of the increased ROS generation ensuing the release of Ag^{+} ions, rather than a high-Z effect [222, 223]. Also iron oxide NPs have shown interesting radiosensitizing effects, which were attributed to the release of Fe^{3+} ions which enhance the production of ROS upon X-ray irradiation [224–226].

Enhanced RT was explored for the local treatment of solid tumors, but in presence of metastatic diseases brachytherapy is preferred. Brachytherapy treatment relies on to systemic injection of radiopharmaceuticals (typically Auger electrons or α- and β-particles) [227–229]. By this approach, ionizing radiation sources wander around the body, hence, achieving tumor specificity is crucial in order to prevent radiotoxicity in healthy organs.

On this regard, several nanocarriers for radioisotopes delivery have been developed, including organic and inorganic nanoformulations of Iodine-131, Yttrium-90 and Rhenium-88 [230–237]. For instance, Tian and co-workers have recently reported the synthesis and *in vivo* investigations of ^{131}I-tagged human serum albumin (^{131}I-HAS) bound to manganese oxide NPs (^{131}I-HAS-MnO_2). Notably, *in vitro* viability assays on 4T1 cells confirmed that ^{131}I-HAS-MnO_2 significantly decrease cells viability, proving that cytotoxicity was induced by accumulation of Iodine-131. Furthermore, *in vivo* brachytherapy was accomplished through tail administration of ^{131}I-HAS-MnO_2, yielding a preferential accumulation at tumor site compared to free ^{131}I-HAS, significantly reducing the tumor growth (Figure 3.13) [238].

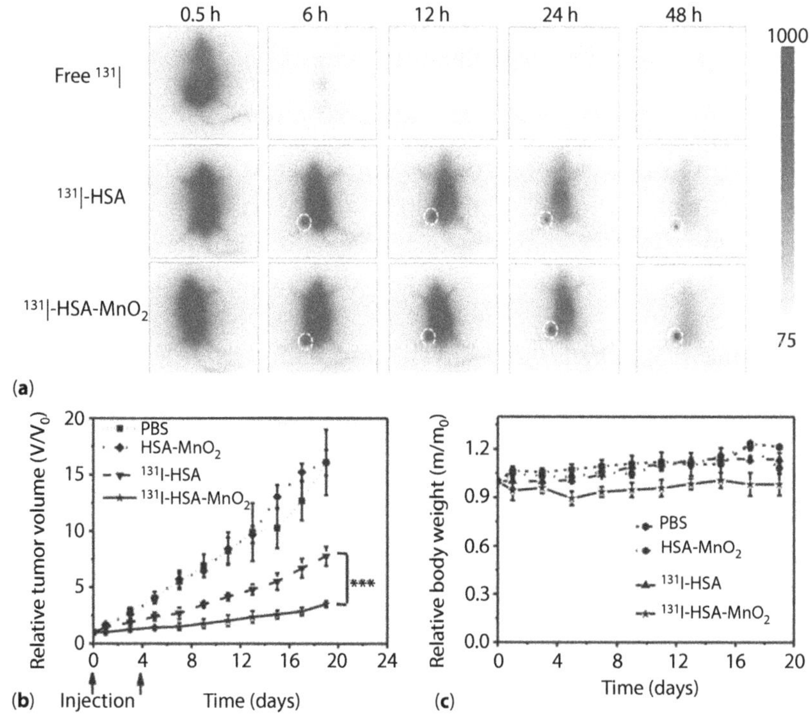

Figure 3.13 (a) *In vivo* gamma imaging after injection of free ^{131}I (up), ^{131}I-HAS (center) and ^{131}I-HAS-MnO_2 (down); (b) relative tumor volume after internal RT treatment and (c) relative mice body weight following RT [238]. Reproduced from [238] with permission of John Wiley & Sons Inc.

References

1. F.K. Richtmyer, F. W. W. The absorption of x-rays by iron, cobalt, nickel and copper. *Phys. Rev.* 22, 539–545, 1923.
2. Danad, I., Fayad, Z. A., Willemink, M. J. & Min, J. K. New applications of cardiac computed tomography: Dual-energy, spectral, and molecular CT imaging. *JACC Cardiovasc. Imaging* 8, 710–723, 2015.
3. Moos, S. I., Van Vemde, D. N. H., Stoker, J. & Bipat, S. Contrast induced nephropathy in patients undergoing intravenous (IV) contrast enhanced computed tomography (CECT) and the relationship with risk factors: A meta-analysis. *Eur. J. Radiol.* 82, e387–e399, 2013.

4. Lee, S. Y. *et al.* A review: Radiographic iodinated contrast media-induced thyroid dysfunction. *J. Clin. Endocrinol. Metab.* 100, 376–383, 2015.
5. Samei, E. *et al.* Micro-CT imaging of breast tumors in rodents using a liposomal, nanoparticle contrast agent. *Int. J. Nanomedicine* 4, 277–282, 2009.
6. Liu, Y. *et al.* A high-performance ytterbium-based nanoparticulate contrast agent for *in vivo* X-ray computed tomography imaging. *Angew. Chemie – Int. Ed.* 51, 1437–1442, 2012.
7. Naha, P. C. *et al.* Gold silver alloy nanoparticles (GSAN): an imaging probe for breast cancer screening with dual-energy mammography or computed tomography. *Nanoscale* 8, 13740–13754, 2016.
8. Caro, C., Dalmases, M., Figuerola, A., García-Martín, M. L. & Leal, M. P. Highly water-stable rare ternary Ag–Au–Se nanocomposites as long blood circulation time X-ray computed tomography contrast agents. *Nanoscale* 9, 7242–7251, 2017.
9. Kim, D., Park, S., Lee, J. H., Jeong, Y. Y. & Jon, S. Antibiofouling polymer-coated gold nanoparticles as a contrast agent for *in vivo* X-ray computed tomography imaging. *J. Am. Chem. Soc.* 129, 7661–5, 2007.
10. Cai, Q. Y. *et al.* Colloidal gold nanoparticles as a blood-pool contrast agent for X-ray computed tomography in mice. *Invest. Radiol.* 42, 797–806, 2007.
11. Cole, L. E., Vargo-Gogola, T. & Roeder, R. K. Bisphosphonate-functionalized gold nanoparticles for contrast-enhanced X-ray detection of breast microcalcifications. *Biomaterials* 35, 2312–2321, 2014.
12. Zhang, Z., Ross, R. D. & Roeder, R. K. Preparation of functionalized gold nanoparticles as a targeted X-ray contrast agent for damaged bone tissue. *Nanoscale* 2, 582, 2010.
13. Hayashi, K., Nakamura, M. & Ishimura, K. Near-Infrared Fluorescent Silica-Coated Gold Nanoparticle Clusters for X-Ray Computed Tomography/Optical Dual Modal Imaging of the Lymphatic System. *Adv. Healthc. Mater.* 2, 756–763, 2013.
14. Wang, Y. *et al.* Label-free Au cluster used for *in vivo* 2D and 3D computed tomography of murine kidneys. *Anal. Chem.* 87, 343–345, 2015.

15. Liu, H. *et al.* Synthesis of PEGylated low generation dendrimer-entrapped gold nanoparticles for CT imaging applications. *Nanoscale* 6, 4521–4526, 2014.
16. Sun, I. C. *et al.* Tumor-targeting gold particles for dual computed tomography/optical cancer imaging. *Angew. Chemie – Int. Ed.* 50, 9348–9351, 2011.
17. Dou, Y. *et al.* Size-Tuning Ionization to Optimize Gold Nanoparticles for Simultaneous Enhanced CT Imaging and Radiotherapy. *ACS Nano* 10, 2536–2548, 2016.
18. Li, Z. *et al.* Graphene Oxide/Ag Nanoparticles Cooperated with Simvastatin as a High Sensitive X-Ray Computed Tomography Imaging Agent for Diagnosis of Renal Dysfunctions. *Adv. Healthc. Mater.* 1700413, 1–11, 2017.
19. Heijblom, M. *et al.* Photoacoustic image patterns of breast carcinoma and comparisons with Magnetic Resonance Imaging and vascular stained histopathology. *Scientific Reports* 5, Article number: 11778, 2015.
20. Peng, D. *et al.* Precise diagnosis in different scenarios using photoacoustic and fluorescence imaging with dual-modality nanoparticles. *Nanoscale* 8, 14480–14488, 2016.
21. Ku, G. *et al.* Copper sulfide nanoparticles as a new class of photoacoustic contrast agent for deep tissue imaging at 1064 nm. *ACS Nano* 6, 7489–7496, 2012.
22. Miao, Q., Lyu, Y., Ding, D. & Pu, K. Semiconducting Oligomer Nanoparticles as an Activatable Photoacoustic Probe with Amplified Brightness for *in vivo* Imaging of pH. *Adv. Mater.* 28, 3662–3668, 2016.
23. De La Zerda, A. *et al.* Carbon nanotubes as photoacoustic molecular imaging agents in living mice. *Nat. Nanotechnol.* 3, 557–562, 2008.
24. Zerda, A. D. La *et al.* Ultrahigh sensitivity carbon nanotube agents for photoacoustic molecular imaging in living mice. *Nano Lett.* 10, 2168–2172, 2010.
25. Jelley, E. E. Spectral Absorption and Fluorescence of Dyes in the Molecular State. *Nature* 138, 1009–1010, 1936.
26. Swiecicki, J.-M. *et al.* How to unveil self-quenched fluorophores and subsequently map the subcellular distribution of exogenous peptides. *Sci. Rep.* 6, 20237, 2016.

27. Liu, R., Tang, J., Xu, Y., Zhou, Y. & Dai, Z. Nano-sized Indocyanine Green J-aggregate as a One-component Theranostic Agent. *Nanotheranostics* 1, 430–439, 2017.
28. Shakiba, M. *et al.* Stable J-aggregation enabled dual photoacoustic and fluorescence nanoparticles for intraoperative cancer imaging. *Nanoscale* 8, 12618–12625, 2016.
29. Bricks, J. L., Slominskii, Y. L., Panas, I. D. & Demchenko, A. P. Fluorescent J-aggregates of cyanine dyes: basic research and applications review. *Methods Appl. Fluoresc.* 6, 12001, 2017.
30. Avigo, C., Cassano, D., Kusmic, C., Voliani, V. & Menichetti, L. Enhanced photoacoustic signal of passion fruit-like nanoarchitectures in a biological environment. *J. Phys. Chem. C* 121, 6955–6961, 2017.
31. Del Guerra, A., Belcari, N. & Bisogni, M. Positron emission tomography: Its 65 years. *Riv. del Nuovo Cim.* 39, 155–223, 2016.
32. Ido *et al.* Labeled 2-deoxy-D-glucose analogs. 18F-labeled 2-deoxy-2-fluoro-D-glucose, 2-deoxy-2-fluoro-D-mannose and 14C-2-deoxy-2-fluoro-D-glucose. *J. Label. Compd. Radiopharm.* 14, 175–183, 1978.
33. Phelps, M. E. Positron emission tomography provides molecular imaging of biological processes. *Proc. Natl. Acad. Sci. U. S. A.* 97, 9226–9233, 2000.
34. Pandya, D. N. *et al.* Zirconium tetraazamacrocycle complexes display extraordinary stability and provide a new strategy for zirconium-89-based radiopharmaceutical development. *Chem. Sci.* 8, 2309–2314, 2017.
35. Wadas, T. J., Wong, E. H., Weisman, G. R. & Anderson, C. J. Coordinating radiometals of copper, gallium, indium, yttrium, and zirconium for PET and SPECT imaging of disease. *Chem. Rev.* 110, 2858–2902, 2010.
36. Spang, P., Herrmann, C. & Roesch, F. Bifunctional Gallium-68 Chelators: Past, Present, and Future. *Semin. Nucl. Med.* 46, 373–394, 2016.
37. Andreozzi, E., Seo, J. W., Ferrara, K. & Louie, A. Novel method to label solid lipid nanoparticles with 64Cu for positron emission tomography imaging. *Bioconjug. Chem.* 22, 808–818, 2011.

38. Liu, T. W. *et al.* Inherently multimodal nanoparticle-driven tracking and real-time delineation of orthotopic prostate tumors and micrometastases. *ACS Nano* 7, 4221–4232, 2013.
39. Sun, X. *et al.* Chelator-free 64Cu-integrated gold nanomaterials for positron emission tomography imaging guided photothermal cancer therapy. *ACS Nano* 8, 8438–8446, 2014.
40. Yang, M. *et al.* Facile Synthesis of ^{64} Cu-Doped Au Nanocages for Positron Emission Tomography Imaging. *ChemNanoMat.* 1–8, 2016.
41. Zhao, Y. *et al.* Copper-64-alloyed gold nanoparticles for cancer imaging: Improved radiolabel stability and diagnostic accuracy. *Angew. Chemie - Int. Ed.* 53, 156–159, 2014.
42. Shaffer, T. M. *et al.* Stable Radiolabeling of Sulfur-Functionalized Silica Nanoparticles with Copper-64. *Nano Lett.* 16, 5601–5604, 2016.
43. Boswell, C. A. *et al.* Comparative *in Vivo* Stability of Copper-64-Labeled Cross-Bridged and Conventional Tetraazamacrocyclic Complexes. *J. Med. Chem.* 47, 1465–1474, 2004.
44. Goel, S., Chen, F., Ehlerding, E. B. & Cai, W. Intrinsically Radiolabeled Nanoparticles: An Emerging Paradigm. *Small* 10, 3825–3830, 2014.
45. Shi, S. *et al.* Chelator-Free Radiolabeling of Nanographene: Breaking the Stereotype of Chelation. *Angew. Chemie - Int. Ed.* 56, 2889–2892, 2017.
46. Boros, E., Bowen, A. M., Josephson, L., Vasdev, N. & Holland, J. P. Chelate-free metal ion binding and heat-induced radiolabeling of iron oxide nanoparticles. *Chem. Sci.* 6, 225–236, 2015.
47. *Nuclear Magnetic Resonance.* 7, (Royal Society of Chemistry, 1978).
48. *Nuclear Magnetic Resonance.* 13, (Royal Society of Chemistry, 1984).
49. Na, H. Bin, Song, I. C. & Hyeon, T. Inorganic nanoparticles for MRI contrast agents. *Adv. Mater.* 21, 2133–2148, 2009.
50. Bottomley 1986 – Review of H T1 and T2 in NMR.pdf.
51. Beall, P. T., Asch, B. B., Chang, D. C., Medina, D. & Hazlewood, C. F. Distinction of normal, preneoplastic, and neoplastic mouse mammary primary cell cultures by water nuclear magnetic resonance relaxation times. *J. Natl. Cancer Inst.* 64, 335–8, 1980.

52. A, B., J, de C., P, D. *et al.* Histological explanation of proton T1 and T2 variations in lung tumors. *Magn. Reson. cancer* 49–51, 1986.
53. Ling, C. R. & Foster, M. A. Changes in NMR relaxation time associated with local inflammatory response. *Phys. Med. Biol.* 27, 853–860, 1982.
54. Braunschweiger, P. G., Schiffer, L. M. & Furmanski, P. 1H-NMR relaxation times and water compartmentalization in experimental tumor models. *Magn. Reson. Imaging* 4, 335–342, 1986.
55. Lauterbur, P. C. & Dias, M. Ferromagnetic Particles as Contrast Agents for Magnetic Resonance Imaging of Liver and Spleen. *Magn. Reson. Med.* 3, 328–330, 1986.
56. Huang, J. *et al.* Effects of Nanoparticle Size on Cellular Uptake and Liver MRI with PVP-Coated Iron Oxide Nanoparticles. *ACS Nano* 4, 7151–7160, 2010.
57. Zhao, Z. *et al.* Octapod iron oxide nanoparticles as high-performance T2 contrast agents for magnetic resonance imaging. *Nat. Commun.* 4, 1–7, 2013.
58. Cheong, S. *et al.* Simple synthesis and functionalization of iron nanoparticles for magnetic resonance imaging. *Angew. Chemie - Int. Ed.* 50, 4206–4209, 2011.
59. Xie, H. *et al.* Lactoferrin-conjugated superparamagnetic iron oxide nanoparticles as a specific MRI contrast agent for detection of brain glioma *in vivo*. *Biomaterials* 32, 495–502, 2011.
60. Andreas, K. *et al.* Highly efficient magnetic stem cell labeling with citrate-coated superparamagnetic iron oxide nanoparticles for MRI tracking. *Biomaterials* 33, 4515–4525, 2012.
61. Wang, Z. *et al.* Active targeting theranostic iron oxide nanoparticles for MRI and magnetic resonance-guided focused ultrasound ablation of lung cancer. *Biomaterials* 127, 25–35, 2017.
62. Evanics, F., Diamente, P. R., Van Veggel, F. C. J. M., Stanisz, G. J. & Prosser, R. S. Water-soluble GdF3 and GdF3/LaF3 nanoparticles – Physical characterization and NMR relaxation properties. *Chem. Mater.* 18, 2499–2505, 2006.
63. Bridot, J.-L. *et al.* Hybrid Gd oxide nanoparticle multimodal contrast agents for *in vivo* imaging. *J. Am. Chem. Soc.* 129, 5076–5084, 2007.

64. Cabrera-García, A. *et al.* Gd-Si Oxide Nanoparticles as Contrast Agents in Magnetic Resonance Imaging. *Nanomaterials* 6, 109, 2016.
65. Park, J. Y. *et al.* Paramagnetic Ultrasmall Gadolinium Oxide Nanoparticles as Advanced T 1 MRI Contrast Agent: Account for Large Longitudinal Relaxivity, Optimal Particle Diameter, and *In Vivo* T 1 MR Images. *ACS Nano* 3, 3663–3669, 2009.
66. Zhou, Z. *et al.* Surface and interfacial engineering of iron oxide nanoplates for highly efficient magnetic resonance angiography. *ACS Nano* 9, 3012–3022, 2015.
67. Shin, T.-H. *et al.* T_1 and T_2 Dual-Mode MRI Contrast Agent for Enhancing Accuracy by Engineered Nanomaterials. *ACS Nano* 8, 3393–3401, 2014.
68. Choi, J. S. *et al.* Self-confirming 'aND' logic nanoparticles for fault-free MRI. *J. Am. Chem. Soc.* 132, 11015–11017, 2010.
69. Li, F. *et al.* Core/shell Fe_3O_4/Gd_2O_3 nanocubes as T_1–T_2 dual modal MRI contrast agents. *Nanoscale* 8, 12826–12833, 2016.
70. Tu, Q. & Chang, C. Diagnostic applications of Raman spectroscopy. *Nanomedicine Nanotechnology, Biol. Med.* 8, 545–558, 2012.
71. Movasaghi, Z., Rehman, S. & Rehman, I. U. Raman spectroscopy of biological tissues. *Appl. Spectrosc. Rev.* 42, 493–541, 2007.
72. Carey, P. R. Raman spectroscopy, the sleeping giant in structural biology, awakes. *J. Biol. Chem.* 274, 26625–26628, 1999.
73. Procházka, M. Surface-Enhanced Raman Spectroscopy. Biological and Medical Physics, *Biomedical Engineering*, 2016. – Bioanalytical, Biomolecular and Medical Applications U6 – http://dx.doi.org/10.1007/978-3-319-23992-7 M4 – Citavi
74. Efremov, E. V., Ariese, F. & Gooijer, C. Achievements in resonance Raman spectroscopy. Review of a technique with a distinct analytical chemistry potential. *Anal. Chim. Acta* 606, 119–134, 2008.
75. Kneipp, J., Kneipp, H. & Kneipp, K. SERS—a single-molecule and nanoscale tool for bioanalytics. *Chem. Soc. Rev.* 37, 1052, 2008.
76. Matousek, P., Towrie, M. & Parker, A. W. Fluorescence background suppression in Raman spectroscopy using combined

Kerr gated and shifted excitation Raman difference techniques. *J. Raman Spectrosc.* 33, 238–242, 2002.

77. Trabesinger, W., Kramer, A., Kreiter, M., Hecht, B. & Wild, U. P. Single-molecule near-field optical energy transfer microscopy. *Appl. Phys. Lett.* 81, 2118–2120, 2002.
78. Anger, P., Bharadwaj, P. & Novotny, L. Enhancement and quenching of single-molecule fluorescence. *Phys. Rev. Lett.* 96, 3–6, 2006.
79. Fleischmann, M., Hendra, P. J. & McQuillan, A. J. Raman spectra of pyridine adsorbed at a silver electrode. *Chem. Phys. Lett.* 26, 163–166, 1974.
80. Nie, S. Probing Single Molecules and Single Nanoparticles by Surface-Enhanced Raman Scattering. *Science (80-.).* 275, 1102–1106, 1997.
81. Le Ru, E. C., Blackie, E., Meyer, M. & Etchegoint, P. G. Surface enhanced raman scattering enhancement factors: A comprehensive study. *J. Phys. Chem. C* 111, 13794–13803, 2007.
82. Bonifacio, A., Cervo, S. & Sergo, V. Label-free surface-enhanced Raman spectroscopy of biofluids : fundamental aspects and diagnostic applications., *Analytical & Bioanalytical Chemistry* 2015.
83. Vo-dinh, T. *et al.* Golden Opportunities in Biomedical Applications. *SERS Nanosensors and Nanoreporters*, 7, 2015.
84. Lane, L. A., Qian, X. & Nie, S. SERS Nanoparticles in Medicine : From Label-Free Detection to Spectroscopic Tagging., *Chem. Rev.* 115 (19), pp. 10489–10529, 2015.
85. Laing, S., Gracie, K., Faulds, K. & Laing, S. Chem Soc Rev Multiplex *in vitro* detection using SERS suspensions as these are relatively easily prepared and are. *Chem. Soc. Rev.* 45, 1901–1918, 2016.
86. Abramczyk, H. & Brozek-pluska, B. Raman Imaging in Biochemical and Biomedical Applications. Diagnosis and Treatment of Breast Cancer., *Chem. Rev.*, 113 (8), pp 5766–5781, 2013.
87. Wang, Z., Zong, S., Wu, L., Zhu, D. & Cui, Y. SERS-Activated Platforms for Immunoassay: Probes, Encoding Methods, and Applications., *Chem. Rev.*, 117 (12), pp 7910–7963, 2017.

88. Samanta, A. *et al.* Ultrasensitive near-infrared Raman reporters for SERS-based *in vivo* cancer detection. *Angew. Chemie – Int. Ed.* 50, 6089–6092, 2011.
89. Dinish, U. S. *et al.* Single molecule with dual function on nanogold: Biofunctionalized construct for *in vivo* photoacoustic imaging and SERS biosensing. *Adv. Funct. Mater.* 25, 2316–2325, 2015.
90. Zhang, Y., Qian, J., Wang, D., Wang, Y. & He, S. Multifunctional gold nanorods with ultrahigh stability and tunability for *in vivo* fluorescence imaging, SERS detection, and photodynamic therapy. *Angew. Chemie – Int. Ed.* 52, 1148–1151, 2013.
91. Yigit, M. V. *et al.* Noninvasive MRI-SERS imaging in living mice using an innately bimodal nanomaterial. *ACS Nano* 5, 1056–1066, 2011.
92. Qian, X. *et al. In vivo* tumor targeting and spectroscopic detection with surface-enhanced Raman nanoparticle tags. *Nat. Biotechnol.* 26, 83–90, 2007.
93. Conde, J., Bao, C., Cui, D., Baptista, P. V. & Tian, F. Antibody-drug gold nanoantennas with Raman spectroscopic fingerprints for *in vivo* tumour theranostics. *J. Control. Release* 183, 87–93, 2014.
94. Tian, F. *et al.* Gold nanostars for efficient *in vitro* and *in vivo* real-time SERS detection and drug delivery via plasmonic-tunable Raman/FTIR imaging. *Biomaterials* 106, 87–97, 2016.
95. Gandra, N. *et al.* Tunable and amplified Raman gold nanoprobes for effective tracking (TARGET): *in vivo* sensing and imaging. *Nanoscale* 8, 8486–8494, 2016.
96. Gilman, A. The initial clinical trial of nitrogen mustard. *Am. J. Surg.* 105, 574–578, 1963.
97. Nygren, P. What is cancer chemotherapy? *Acta Oncol* 40, 166–174, 2001.
98. Muggia, F. Platinum compounds 30 years after the introduction of cisplatin: Implications for the treatment of ovarian cancer. *Gynecol. Oncol.* 112, 275–281, 2009.
99. Shaloam, D. & Tchounwou, P. B. Cisplatin in cancer therapy: Molecular mechanisms of action. *Eur. J. Pharmacol.* 740, 364–378, 2014.

100. Löwenberg, B. *et al.* Cytarabine Dose for Acute Myeloid Leukemia. *N. Engl. J. Med.* 364, 1027–1036, 2011.
101. Mini, E., Nobili, S., Caciagli, B., Landini, I. & Mazzei, T. Cellular pharmacology of gemcitabine. *Ann. Oncol.* 17, 7–12, 2006.
102. Gottesman, M. M. Mechanisms of Cancer Drug Resistance. *Annu. Rev. Med.* 53, 615–627, 2002.
103. Dumontet, C. & Jordan, M. A. Microtubule-binding agents: a dynamic field of cancer therapeutics. *Nat. Rev. Drug Discov.* 9, 897–897, 2010.
104. Side Effects of Chemotherapy. at <https://www.cancer.net/navigating-cancer-care/how-cancer-treated/chemotherapy/side-effects-chemotherapy>
105. Gottesman, M. M. Mechanisms of Cancer Drug Resistance. *Annu. Rev. Med.* 53, 615–627, 2002.
106. Gregoriadis, G. Drug entrapment in liposomes. *FEBS Lett.* 36, 292–296, 1973.
107. Northfelt, D. W. *et al.* Doxorubicin Encapsulated in Liposomes Containing Surface-Bound Polyethylene Glycol: Pharmacokinetics, Tumor Localization, and Safety in Patients with AIDS-Related Kaposi's Sarcoma. *J. Clin. Pharmacol.* 36, 55–63, 1996.
108. Harrington, K. J. *et al.* Phase I-II study of pegylated liposomal cisplatin (SPI-077) in patients with inoperable head and neck cancer. *Ann. Oncol. Off. J. Eur. Soc. Med. Oncol.* 12, 493–6, 2001.
109. Sharma, A. *et al.* Activity of paclitaxel liposome formulations against human ovarian tumor xenografts. *Int. J. Cancer* 71, 103–107, 1997.
110. Kato, M. Overview of the state-of-the-art liposomal drug analysis using high-performance liquid chromatography. *Appl. Spectrosc. Rev.* 4928, 1–11, 2017.
111. Ghosh, P., Han, G., De, M., Kim, C. K. & Rotello, V. M. Gold nanoparticles in delivery applications. *Adv. Drug Deliv. Rev.* 60, 1307–1315, 2008.
112. Mura, S., Nicolas, J. & Couvreur, P. Stimuli-responsive nanocarriers for drug delivery. *Nat. Mater.* 12, 991–1003, 2013.
113. Kim, C., Ghosh, P. & Rotello, V. M. Multimodal drug delivery using gold nanoparticles. *Nanoscale* 1, 61, 2009.

114. Yavuz, M. S. *et al.* Gold nanocages covered by smart polymers for controlled release with near-infrared light. *Nat. Mater.* 8, 935–939, 2009.
115. Chang, Y. T. *et al.* Near-Infrared light-responsive intracellular drug and sirna release using au nanoensembles with oligonucleotide-capped silica shell. *Adv. Mater.* 24, 3309–3314, 2012.
116. You, J. *et al.* Effective photothermal chemotherapy using doxorubicin-loaded gold nanospheres that target EphB4 receptors in tumors. *Cancer Res.* 72, 4777–4786, 2012.
117. Voliani, V. *et al.* Multiphoton molecular photorelease in click-chemistry-functionalized gold nanoparticles. *Small* 7, 3271–5, 2011.
118. Zhu, H. *et al.* Co-delivery of chemotherapeutic drugs with vitamin E TPGS by porous PLGA nanoparticles for enhanced chemotherapy against multi-drug resistance. *Biomaterials* 35, 2391–2400, 2014.
119. Guo, J. *et al.* Aptamer-functionalized PEG-PLGA nanoparticles for enhanced anti-glioma drug delivery. *Biomaterials* 32, 8010–8020, 2011.
120. Sun, B., Ranganathan, B. & Feng, S. S. Multifunctional poly(d,l-lactide-co-glycolide)/montmorillonite (PLGA/MMT) nanoparticles decorated by Trastuzumab for targeted chemotherapy of breast cancer. *Biomaterials* 29, 475–486, 2008.
121. Bowerman, C. J. *et al.* Docetaxel-loaded PLGA nanoparticles improve efficacy in taxane-resistant triple-negative breast cancer. *Nano Lett.* 17, 242–248, 2017.
122. Xu, X. *et al.* Enhancing tumor cell response to chemotherapy through nanoparticle-mediated codelivery of siRNA and cisplatin prodrug. *Proc. Natl. Acad. Sci. U.S.A.* 110, 18638–18643, 2013.
123. Tian, J. *et al.* Co-delivery of paclitaxel and cisplatin with biocompatible PLGA–PEG nanoparticles enhances chemoradiotherapy in non-small cell lung cancer models. *J. Mater. Chem. B* 5, 6049–6057, 2017.
124. Croissant, J. G., Fatieiev, Y. & Khashab, N. M. Degradability and Clearance of Silicon, Organosilica, Silsesquioxane, Silica Mixed Oxide, and Mesoporous Silica Nanoparticles. *Adv. Mater.* 29, 2017.

125. Cheng, W. *et al.* pH-Sensitive Delivery Vehicle Based on Folic Acid-Conjugated Polydopamine-Modified Mesoporous Silica Nanoparticles for Targeted Cancer Therapy. *ACS Appl. Mater. Interfaces* 9, 18462–18473, 2017.
126. Kienzle, A. *et al.* Dendritic Mesoporous Silica Nanoparticles for pH-Stimuli-Responsive Drug Delivery of TNF-Alpha. *Adv. Healthc. Mater.* 6, 1–9, 2017.
127. Han, W., Chilkoti, A. & López, G. P. Self-assembled hybrid elastin-like polypeptide/silica nanoparticles enable triggered drug release. *Nanoscale* 9, 6178–6186, 2017.
128. Palanikumar, L. *et al.* Spatiotemporally and Sequentially-Controlled Drug Release from Polymer Gatekeeper–Hollow Silica Nanoparticles. *Sci. Rep.* 7, 46540, 2017.
129. Liu, Q. *et al.* Dacarbazine-Loaded Hollow Mesoporous Silica Nanoparticles Grafted with Folic Acid for Enhancing Antimetastatic Melanoma Response. *ACS Appl. Mater. Interfaces* 9, 21673–21687, 2017.
130. Shen, J. *et al.* Multi-step encapsulation of chemotherapy and gene silencing agents in functionalized mesoporous silica nanoparticles. *Nanoscale* 9, 5329–5341, 2017.
131. Zhang, Q., Shen, C., Zhao, N. & Xu, F. J. Redox-Responsive and Drug-Embedded Silica Nanoparticles with Unique Self-Destruction Features for Efficient Gene/Drug Codelivery. *Adv. Funct. Mater.* 27, 2017.
132. Dai, Y. *et al.* 808 Nm Near-Infrared Light Controlled Dual-Drug Release and Cancer Therapy *in vivo* By Upconversion Mesoporous Silica Nanostructures. *J. Mater. Chem. B* 1–15, 2017.
133. Mallory, M., Gogineni, E., Jones, G. C., Greer, L. & Simone, C. B. Therapeutic hyperthermia: The old, the new, and the upcoming. *Crit. Rev. Oncol. Hematol.* 97, 56–64, 2016.
134. Barlogie, B., Corry, P. M. & Drewinko, B. *In Vitro* Thermochemotherapy of Human Colon Cancer Cells with cis-Dichlorodiammineplatinum(ll) and Mitomycin C'. *Cancer Res.* 40, 1165–1168, 1980.
135. Olav Dahl, M. D. Hyperthermic potentiation of doxorubicin and 4' -epi-doxorubicin in a transplantable neurogenic rat tumor (BT,A) in BD IX rats. *Int. J. Radiat. Oncol. Biol. Phys.* 9, 203–207, 1982.

136. Cividalli D.sc, A., Cruciani, G., Livdi, E., Pasqualetti, P. & Tirindelli Danesi, D. Hyperthermia enhances the response of paclitaxel and radiation in a mouse adenocarcinoma. *Int. J. Radiat. Oncol. Biol. Phys.* 44, 407–412, 1999.
137. Vertrees, R. A. *et al.* Synergistic interaction of hyperthermia and gemcitabine in lung cancer. *Cancer Biol. Ther.* 4, 1144–1153, 2005.
138. Robinson, J., Wizenberg, M. & McCready, W. Combined hyperthermia and radiation suggest an alternative to heavy particle therapy for reduced oxygen enhancement ratios. *Nature* 251, 521–522, 1974.
139. Oei, A. L., Vriend, L. E. M., Crezee, J., Franken, N. A. P. & Krawczyk, P. M. Effects of hyperthermia on DNA repair pathways: one treatment to inhibit them all. *Radiat. Oncol.* 10, 165, 2015.
140. Mikheeva, S. *et al.* Alterations in gene expression induced in day-9 mouse embryos exposed to hyperthermia (HS) or 4-hydroperoxycyclophosphamide (4CP): Analysis using cDNA microarrays. *Toxicol. Sci.* 79, 345–359, 2004.
141. Furukawa, K., Kikusato, M., Kamizono, T., Yoshida, H. & Toyomizu, M. Possible Involvement of Mitochondrial Reactive Oxygen Species Production in Protein Degradation Induced by Heat Stress in Avian Muscle Cells., 2015.
142. Welch, W. I. & Suhan, J. P. Morphological study of the mammalian stress response: Characterization of changes in cytoplasmic organelles, cytoskeleton, and nucleoli, and appearance of intranuclear actin filaments in rat fibroblasts after heat-shock treatment. *J. Cell Biol.* 101, 1198–1211, 1985.
143. Calderwood, S. K., Theriault, J. R. & Gong, J. How is the immune response affected by hyperthermia and heat shock proteins? *Int. J. Hyperth.* 21, 713–716, 2005.
144. Richter, K., Haslbeck, M. & Buchner, J. The Heat Shock Response: Life on the Verge of Death. *Mol. Cell* 40, 253–266, 2010.
145. van der Zee, J. Heating the patient: A promising approach? *Ann. Oncol.* 13, 1173–1184, 2002.
146. Kregel, K. C. & Sieck, G. C. Heat shock proteins: modifying factors in physiological stress responses and acquired thermotolerance. *J. Appl. Physiol.* 89, 1253–1254, 2002.

147. Jaque, D. *et al.* Nanoparticles for photothermal therapies. *Nanoscale* 6, 9494–9530, 2014.
148. Huang, X., El-Sayed, I. H., Qian, W. & El-Sayed, M. A. Cancer cell imaging and photothermal therapy in the near-infrared region by using gold nanorods. *J. Am. Chem. Soc.* 128, 2115–2120, 2006.
149. Li, J. L., Day, D. & Gu, M. Ultra-low energy threshold for cancer photothermal therapy using transferrin-conjugated gold nanorods. *Adv. Mater.* 20, 3866–3871, 2008.
150. Choi, W. Il *et al.* Tumor regression *in vivo* by photothermal therapy based on gold-nanorod-loaded, functional nanocarriers. *ACS Nano* 5, 1995–2003, 2011.
151. Tsai, M. F. *et al.* Au nanorod design as light-absorber in the first and second biological near-infrared windows for *in vivo* photothermal therapy. *ACS Nano* 7, 5330–5342, 2013.
152. Shen, S. *et al.* Targeting mesoporous silica-encapsulated gold nanorods for chemo-photothermal therapy with near-infrared radiation. *Biomaterials* 34, 3150–3158, 2013.
153. Wang, B. *et al.* Rose-bengal-conjugated gold nanorods for invivo photodynamic and photothermal oral cancer therapies. *Biomaterials* 35, 1954–1966, 2014.
154. Yang, M. *et al.* Mitomycin C-treated human-induced pluripotent stem cells as a safe delivery system of gold nanorods for targeted photothermal therapy of gastric cancer. *Nanoscale* 9, 334–340, 2017.
155. Zhao, X., Yang, C.-X., Chen, L.-G. & Yan, X.-P. Dual-stimuli responsive and reversibly activatable theranostic nanoprobe for precision tumor-targeting and fluorescence-guided photothermal therapy. *Nat. Commun.* 8, 14998, 2017.
156. Liu, H. *et al.* Multifunctional gold nanoshells on silica nanorattles: A platform for the combination of photothermal therapy and chemotherapy with low systemic toxicity. *Angew. Chemie - Int. Ed.* 50, 891–895, 2011.
157. Gobin, A. M. *et al.* Near-infrared resonant nanoshells for combined optical imaging and photothermal cancer therapy. *Nano Lett.* 7, 1929–1934, 2007.
158. Wang, S. *et al.* Single continuous wave laser induced photodynamic/plasmonic photothermal therapy using

photosensitizer-functionalized gold nanostars. *Adv. Mater.* 25, 3055–3061, 2013.

159. Qiu, P. *et al.* Tuning photothermal properties of gold nanodendrites for *in vivo* cancer therapy within a wide near infrared range by simply controlling their degree of branching. *Biomaterials* 104, 138–144, 2016.
160. Chen, J. *et al.* Immuno gold nanocages with tailored optical properties for targeted photothermal destruction of cancer cells. *Nano Lett.* 7, 1318–1322, 2007.
161. Wu, X. *et al.* High-photoluminescence-yield gold nanocubes: For cell imaging and photothermal therapy. *ACS Nano* 4, 113–120, 2010.
162. Ayala-Orozco, C. *et al.* Au nanomatryoshkas as efficient near-infrared photothermal transducers for cancer treatment: Benchmarking against nanoshells. *ACS Nano* 8, 6372–6381, 2014.
163. Zhu, X. M., Wan, H. Y., Jia, H., Liu, L. & Wang, J. Porous Pt Nanoparticles with High Near-Infrared Photothermal Conversion Efficiencies for Photothermal Therapy. *Adv. Healthc. Mater.* 5, 3165–3172, 2016.
164. Fang, W. *et al.* Pd nanosheet-covered hollow mesoporous silica nanoparticles as a platform for the chemo-photothermal treatment of cancer cells. *Small* 8, 3816–3822, 2012.
165. He, W. *et al.* Plasmonic titanium nitride nanoparticles for *in vivo* photoacoustic tomography imaging and photothermal cancer therapy. *Biomaterials* 132, 37–47, 2017.
166. Markovic, Z. M. *et al.* *In vitro* comparison of the photothermal anticancer activity of graphene nanoparticles and carbon nanotubes. *Biomaterials* 32, 1121–1129, 2011.
167. Moon, H. K., Lee, S. H. & Choi, H. C. *In vivo* near-infrared mediated tumor destruction by photothermal effect of carbon nanotubes. *ACS Nano* 3, 3707–3713, 2009.
168. Yang, K. *et al.* Graphene in mice: Ultrahigh *in vivo* tumor uptake and efficient photothermal therapy. *Nano Lett.* 10, 3318–3323, 2010.
169. Zhang, W. *et al.* Synergistic effect of chemo-photothermal therapy using PEGylated graphene oxide. *Biomaterials* 32, 8555–8561, 2011.

170. Yu, N. *et al.* Dynamically tuning near-infrared-induced photothermal performances of TiO_2 nanocrystals by Nb doping for imaging-guided photothermal therapy of tumors. *Nanoscale* 9, 9148–9159, 2017.
171. Hessel, C. M. *et al.* Copper selenide nanocrystals for photothermal therapy. *Nano Lett.* 11, 2560–2566, 2011.
172. Yu, X., Yang, K., Chen, X. & Li, W. Black hollow silicon oxide nanoparticles as highly efficient photothermal agents in the second near-infrared window for *in vivo* cancer therapy. *Biomaterials* 143, 120–129, 2017.
173. Cheng, L., Yang, K., Chen, Q. & Liu, Z. Organic stealth nanoparticles for highly effective *in vivo* near-infrared photothermal therapy of cancer. *ACS Nano* 6, 5605–5613, 2012.
174. Yang, J. *et al.* Convertible organic nanoparticles for near-infrared photothermal ablation of cancer cells. *Angew. Chemie - Int. Ed.* 50, 441–444, 2011.
175. Yang, K. *et al. In vitro* and *in vivo* near-infrared photothermal therapy of cancer using polypyrrole organic nanoparticles. *Adv. Mater.* 24, 5586–5592, 2012.
176. Zheng, M. *et al.* Single-step assembly of DOX/ICG loaded lipid-polymer nanoparticles for highly effective chemo-photothermal combination therapy. *ACS Nano* 7, 2056–2067, 2013.
177. Ramprasad, R., Zurcher, P., Petras, M., Miller, M. & Renaud, P. Magnetic properties of metallic ferromagnetic nanoparticle composites. *J. Appl. Phys.* 96, 519–529, 2004.
178. Dennis, C. L. & Ivkov, R. Physics of heat generation using magnetic nanoparticles for hyperthermia. *Int. J. Hyperth.* 29, 715–729, 2013.
179. Stoner, E. C. and W. E. P. A mechanism of magnetic hysteresis in heterogeneous alloys. 826, 1948.
180. Rosensweig, R. E. E. Heating magnetic fluid with alternating magnetic field. *J. Magn. Magn. Mater.* 252, 370–374, 2002.
181. Gilchrist, R. K. *et al.* Selective Inductive Heating of Lymph Nodes. *Ann. Surg.* 146, 596–606, 1957.
182. Landi, G. T. Role of dipolar interaction in magnetic hyperthermia. *Phys. Rev. B - Condens. Matter Mater. Phys.* 89, 1–6, 2014.

183. Mehdaoui, B. *et al.* Increase of magnetic hyperthermia efficiency due to dipolar interactions in low-anisotropy magnetic nanoparticles: Theoretical and experimental results. *Phys. Rev. B - Condens. Matter Mater. Phys.* 87, 1–10, 2013.
184. Haase, C. & Nowak, U. Role of dipole-dipole interactions for hyperthermia heating of magnetic nanoparticle ensembles. *Phys. Rev. B - Condens. Matter Mater. Phys.* 85, 2–6, 2012.
185. Dennis, C. L. *et al.* Nearly complete regression of tumors via collective behavior of magnetic nanoparticles in hyperthermia. *Nanotechnology* 20, 395103, 2009.
186. Andreu, I., Natividad, E., Solozábal, L. & Roubeau, O. Nano-objects for addressing the control of nanoparticle arrangement and performance in magnetic hyperthermia. *ACS Nano* 9, 1408–1419, 2015.
187. Espinosa, A. *et al.* Can magneto-plasmonic nanohybrids efficiently combine photothermia with magnetic hyperthermia? *Nanoscale* 7, 18872–18877, 2015.
188. Ding, Q. *et al.* Shape-controlled fabrication of magnetite silver hybrid nanoparticles with high performance magnetic hyperthermia. *Biomaterials* 124, 35–46, 2017.
189. Hervault, A. *et al.* Doxorubicin loaded dual pH- and thermo-responsive magnetic nanocarrier for combined magnetic hyperthermia and targeted controlled drug delivery applications. *Nanoscale* 8, 12152–12161, 2016.
190. Chen, X. *et al.* Magnetic silica nanotubes: Synthesis, drug release, and feasibility for magnetic hyperthermia. *ACS Appl. Mater. Interfaces* 4, 2303–2309, 2012.
191. Qu, Y. *et al.* Enhanced synergism of thermo-chemotherapy by combining highly efficient magnetic hyperthermia with magnetothermally-facilitated drug release. *Nanoscale* 6, 2014.
192. Lu, F., Popa, A., Zhou, S., Zhu, J.-J. & Samia, A. C. S. Iron oxide-loaded hollow mesoporous silica nanocapsules for controlled drug release and hyperthermia. *Chem. Commun.* 49, 11436, 2013.
193. Sadhukha, T., Wiedmann, T. S. & Panyam, J. Inhalable magnetic nanoparticles for targeted hyperthermia in lung cancer therapy. *Biomaterials* 34, 5163–5171, 2013.

194. Li, T. J. *et al. In vivo* anti-cancer efficacy of magnetite nanocrystal – based system using locoregional hyperthermia combined with 5-fluorouracil chemotherapy. *Biomaterials* 34, 7873–7883, 2013.
195. Zhao, Q. *et al.* Magnetic nanoparticle-based hyperthermia for head & neck cancer in mouse models. *Theranostics* 2, 113–121, 2012.
196. Liu, X. L. *et al.* Synthesis of Ferromagnetic Fe0.6Mn0.4O Nanoflowers as a New Class of Magnetic Theranostic Platform for *In Vivo* T1–T2 Dual-Mode Magnetic Resonance Imaging and Magnetic Hyperthermia Therapy. *Adv. Healthc. Mater.* 5, 2092–2104, 2016.
197. Smith, S. & Prewett, S. Principles of chemotherapy and radiotherapy. *Obstet. Gynaecol. Reprod. Med.* 1–7, 2017.
198. Cooper, D. R., Bekah, D. & Nadeau, J. L. Gold nanoparticles and their alternatives for radiation therapy enhancement. 2, 1–13, 2014.
199. Kobayashi, K., Usami, N., Porcel, E., Lacombe, S. & Sech, C. Le. Enhancement of radiation effect by heavy elements. *Mutat. Res. Mutat. Res.* 704, 123–131, 2010.
200. Carter, J. D., Cheng, N. N., Qu, Y., Suarez, G. D. & Guo, T. *Nanoscale Energy Deposition by X-ray Absorbing Nanostructures. J. Physical Chemistry B*, (40): 11622–11625, 2007.
201. Jain, S. *et al.* Cell-Specific Radiosensitization By Gold Nanoparticles At Megavoltage Radiation Energies. 79, 531–539, 2011.
202. Ferrero, V., Dalmasso, F., Gobbato, A. & Strigari, L. Targeted dose enhancement in radiotherapy for breast cancer using gold nanoparticles, part 1 : A radiobiological model study.
203. Ma, N. *et al.* Shape-Dependent Radiosensitization Effect of Gold Nanostructures in Cancer Radiotherapy: Comparison of Gold Nanoparticles, *ACS Appl. Mater. Interfaces*, 9 (15), pp 13037–13048, 2017.
204. Bhattarai, S. R. *et al.* Gold nanotriangles: scale up and X-ray radiosensitization effects in mice. *Nanoscale* 9, 5085–5093, 2017.
205. Ma, N. *et al.* Enhanced Radiosensitization of Gold Nanospikes via Hyperthermia in Combined Cancer Radiation and Photothermal Therapy. *ACS Appl. Mater. Interfaces* 8, 28480–28494, 2016.

206. Zhang, P. *et al.* Enhanced Radiation Therapy with Multilayer Microdisks Containing Radiosensitizing Gold Nanoparticles. *ACS Appl. Mater. Interfaces* 7, 4518–4524, 2015.
207. Wolfe, T. *et al.* Targeted gold nanoparticles enhance sensitization of prostate tumors to megavoltage radiation therapy *in vivo*. *Nanomedicine Nanotechnology, Biol. Med.* 11, 1277–1283, 2015.
208. Zhang, X.-D. *et al.* Size-dependent radiosensitization of PEG-coated gold nanoparticles for cancer radiation therapy. *Biomaterials* 33, 6408–6419, 2012.
209. Chang, M.-Y. *et al.* Increased apoptotic potential and dose-enhancing effect of gold nanoparticles in combination with single-dose clinical electron beams on tumor-bearing mice. *Cancer Sci.* 99, 1479–1484, 2008.
210. Joh, D. Y. *et al.* Selective Targeting of Brain Tumors with Gold Nanoparticle-Induced Radiosensitization. *PLoS One* 8, e62425, 2013.
211. Wason, M. S. *et al.* Sensitization of pancreatic cancer cells to radiation by cerium oxide nanoparticle-induced ROS production. *Nanomedicine Nanotechnology, Biol. Med.* 9, 558–569, 2013.
212. Briggs, A. *et al.* Cerium oxide nanoparticles: influence of the high-Z component revealed on radioresistant 9L cell survival under X-ray irradiation. *Nanomedicine Nanotechnology, Biol. Med.* 9, 1098–1105, 2013.
213. Chen, F. *et al.* Enhancement of radiotherapy by ceria nanoparticles modified with neogambogic acid in breast cancer cells. *Int. J. Nanomedicine* 4957, 10(1), pp. 4957—4969, 2015.
214. Maggiorella, L. *et al.* Nanoscale radiotherapy with hafnium oxide nanoparticles. *Futur. Oncol.* 8, 1167–1181, 2012.
215. Mao, F. *et al.* Ultrasmall Biocompatible Bi 2 Se 3 Nanodots for Multimodal Imaging-Guided Synergistic Radiophotothermal Therapy against Cancer. *ACS Nano* 10, 11145–11155, 2016.
216. Mowat, P. *et al.* *In Vitro* Radiosensitizing Effects of Ultrasmall Gadolinium Based Particles on Tumour Cells. *J. Nanosci. Nanotechnol.* 11, 7833–7839, 2011.
217. Sancey, L. *et al.* The use of theranostic gadolinium-based nanoprobes to improve radiotherapy efficacy. *Br. J. Radiol.* 87, 20140134, 2014.

218. Zhang, D. G., Feygelman, V., Moros, E. G., Latifi, K. & Zhang, G. G. Monte Carlo Study of Radiation Dose Enhancement by Gadolinium in Megavoltage and High Dose Rate Radiotherapy. *PLoS One* 9, e109389, 2014.
219. Lu, R. Egg white-mediated green synthesis of silver nanoparticles with excellent biocompatibility and enhanced radiation effects on cancer cells. *Int. J. Nanomedicine* 7, pp. 2101–2107, 2012.
220. Liu, P. *et al.* Silver nanoparticles: A novel radiation sensitizer for glioma? *Nanoscale* 5, 11829, 2013.
221. Liu, P. *et al.* Silver nanoparticles outperform gold nanoparticles in radiosensitizing U251 cells *in vitro* and in an intracranial mouse model of glioma. *Int. J. Nanomedicine* 11, 5003–5014, 2016.
222. Cortese-Krott, M. M. *et al.* Silver ions induce oxidative stress and intracellular zinc release in human skin fibroblasts. *Free Radic. Biol. Med.* 47, 1570–1577, 2009.
223. De Matteis, V. *et al.* Negligible particle-specific toxicity mechanism of silver nanoparticles: The role of Ag+ ion release in the cytosol. *Nanomedicine Nanotechnology, Biol. Med.* 11, 731–739, 2015.
224. Huang, G. *et al.* Superparamagnetic iron oxide nanoparticles: Amplifying ros stress to improve anticancer drug efficacy. *Theranostics* 3, 116–126, 2013.
225. Meidanchi, A. *et al.* ZnFe2O4 nanoparticles as radiosensitizers in radiotherapy of human prostate cancer cells. *Mater. Sci. Eng. C* 46, 394–399, 2015.
226. Hauser, A. K. *et al.* Targeted iron oxide nanoparticles for the enhancement of radiation therapy. *Biomaterials* 105, 127–135, 2016.
227. Wernicke, A. G. *et al.* Cesium-131 brachytherapy for recurrent brain metastases: durable salvage treatment for previously irradiated metastatic disease. *J. Neurosurg.* 126, 1212–1219, 2017.
228. Denecke, T. & Lopez Hänninen, E. Brachytherapy of liver metastases. *Recent Results Cancer Res.* 177, 95–104, 2008.
229. Sharma, D. N. *et al.* High-dose-rate interstitial brachytherapy for liver metastases: first study from India. *J. Contemp. Brachytherapy* 2, 70–75, 2013.

230. Song, G., Cheng, L., Chao, Y., Yang, K. & Liu, Z. Emerging Nanotechnology and Advanced Materials for Cancer Radiation Therapy. *Adv. Mater.* 29, 1–26, 2017.
231. Chen, L. *et al.* Radionuclide 131I labeled reduced graphene oxide for nuclear imaging guided combined radio- and photothermal therapy of cancer. *Biomaterials* 66, 21–28, 2015.
232. Zhu, J. *et al.* Radionuclide 131 I-labeled multifunctional dendrimers for targeted SPECT imaging and radiotherapy of tumors. *Nanoscale* 7, 18169–18178, 2015.
233. Zhao, L. *et al.* Chlorotoxin-Conjugated Multifunctional Dendrimers Labeled with Radionuclide 131 I for Single Photon Emission Computed Tomography Imaging and Radiotherapy of Gliomas. *ACS Appl. Mater. Interfaces* 7, 19798–19808, 2015.
234. Buckway, B., Frazier, N., Gormley, A. J., Ray, A. & Ghandehari, H. Gold nanorod-mediated hyperthermia enhances the efficacy of HPMA copolymer-90Y conjugates in treatment of prostate tumors. *Nucl. Med. Biol.* 41, 282–289, 2014.
235. Radović, M. *et al.* Preparation and *in vivo* evaluation of multifunctional 90 Y-labeled magnetic nanoparticles designed for cancer therapy. *J. Biomed. Mater. Res. Part A* 103, 126–134, 2015.
236. Chang, C.-M. *et al.* 188Re-Liposome Can Induce Mitochondrial Autophagy and Reverse Drug Resistance for Ovarian Cancer: From Bench Evidence to Preliminary Clinical Proof-of-Concept. *Int. J. Mol. Sci.* 18, 903, 2017.
237. Chao, Y. *et al.* Rhenium-188 Labeled Tungsten Disulfide Nanoflakes for Self-Sensitized, Near-Infrared Enhanced Radioisotope Therapy. *Small* 12, 3967–3975, 2016.
238. Tian, L. *et al.* Albumin-Templated Manganese Dioxide Nanoparticles for Enhanced Radioisotope Therapy. *Small* 13, 1700640, 2017.

4

Interactions of Nanomaterials with Biological Systems

4.1 Cellular Level (*in vitro*)

4.1.1 Cellular Uptake and Intracellular Fate

Internalization of macromolecules inside cells occurs through endocytosis. However, depending on the size, charge and degree of hydrophobicity, the cellular uptake of nutrients, proteins, signaling factors and other important biomolecules, can follow diverse pathways. This is also true for nanomaterials. The two main routes by which macromolecules and nanomaterials diffuse inside cells from the extracellular *milieu* are phagocytosis and pinocytosis.

Phagocytic uptake is the main mechanism through which molecules or materials whose size exceeds some hundreds of nm are internalized by cells. Indeed, it is generally accepted that phagocytosis occurs mainly for materials above 500 nm, though some groups have reported phagocytic uptake of smaller nanoparticles [1]. During phagocytosis, nanomaterials in physical contact with cells are engulfed and drawn inward within the cytoplasm through invagination of plasma membrane into vesicles called phagosome. Phagocytosis is a very specific uptake pathway, since it occurs through recognizing binding proteins. It is the main mechanism employed by immune system to provide clearance of pathogens from the body through specialized phagocytic cells, called macrophages, which are capable of engulfing particles even bigger than their own volume.

Pinocytosis is an internalization mechanism that takes place through uptake of fluids containing solutes (*e.g.* macromolecules or nanomaterials). Pinocytosis is classified in four subroutes which are either non-specific (macropinocytosis and adsorptive pinocytosis) or specific receptor-mediated pathways.

During macropinocytosis, a huge amount of extracellular material is internalized non-specifically through plasma membrane protrusion and retraction initiated by actin filaments (Figure 4.1). Fluids and solutes are internalized into large vesicles called macropinosomes. Macropinosomes are different

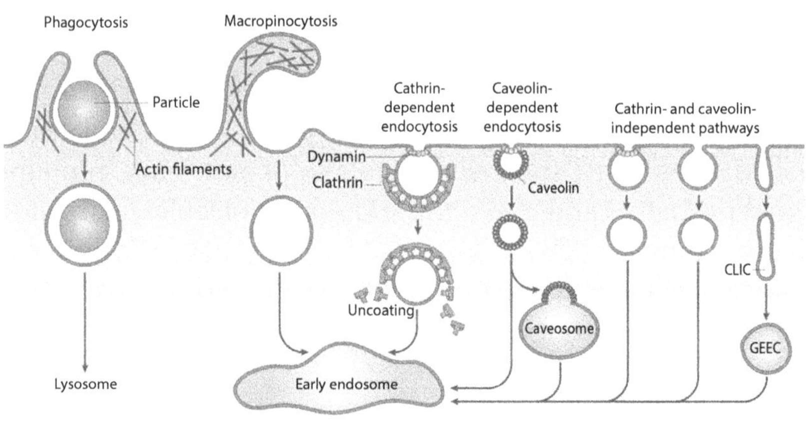

Figure 4.1 Scheme of the possible endocytic pathways and intracellular fate following internalization. Reproduced with permission from [2]. Reproduced with permission from [194]. Copyright 2007 Springer Nature.

from other endocytic vesicles owing to their size, which can reach 5 μm in diameter. Although non-specific, macropinocytosis internalization route is of relevant biological interest since it is often triggered by growth factors stimulation, such as tumor-promoting factors. Because it requires cytoskeleton reorganization, it has been implicated in cell motility during tumor progression [3].

Adsorptive pinocytosis is another non-specific endocytic pathway which is peculiar for cationic molecules or particles. Positively charged particles adhere on cell surface by electrostatic interaction with negatively charged polar heads of phospholipids constituting the plasma membrane, resulting in their non-specific internalization by small vesicles. Adsorptive pinocytosis differs from non-adsorptive pinocytosis because in the latter mechanism molecules or particles are internalized in the fluid phase without adhering to the plasma membrane [4].

Clathrin-mediated endocytosis is the main pathway through which specific internalization of macromolecules occurs in eukaryotes. This endocytic route is related to specific ligands recognized by receptors on plasma membrane. The ligand-receptor complex diffuses through the plasma membrane toward the cytoplasm and be retained in a pit coated by clathrin proteins. Once the pit is mature, it undergoes pinch off from the membrane owing to the action of dynamin proteins. Thus, the clathrin-coated vesicles diffuse in the cytosol. It is worth to note that clathrin-mediated endocytic pathway is size-dependent; the accepted upper size limit of nanomaterials is 200 nm [5]. One of the most interesting examples of clathrin-mediated endocytosis pathway is related to the iron-binding protein transferrin. In the last decades, it has been extensively investigated as a promising protein to enable active targeted drug delivery to cancer cells overexpressing transferrin receptors (TfR) [6]. The most employed strategy to exploit transferrin-mediated endocytosis involve the coating of nanomaterials with antibodies against TfR or transferrin conjugates [7, 8].

Recently, a smart approach to exploit TfR targeting relies on the development of short peptides able to bind transferrin for an endogenous transferrin coating of nanomaterials, in order to modulate the protein corona formation.

On this regard, Santi *et al.* have recently reported the rational design and implementation of a transferrin-binding peptide that anchors the protein on suitable pockets without perturbing the TfR active site for iron docking, leaving unaltered the transferrin biological functionalities [9]. This peptide was employed as coating on the surface of gold NPs and has demonstrated: i) an efficient transferrin binding, ii) a reduction of aspecific protein adsorption on nanoparticles surface, and iii) an enhanced clathrin mediated endocytosis of gold NPs towards human pancreatic cancer cells.

Several receptor-mediated endocytic pathways are clathrin-independents. Among them, caveolin-mediated endocytosis is the most promising for drug delivery applications. Caveolae were firstly described in the early 1950s as omega-shaped plasma membrane pits enriched in cholesterol and sphingolipids. Caveolae pathway can be employed by materials showing a maximum average diameter of 100 nm. Caveolae are mainly constituted by caveolin-1 (Cav-1) proteins. Cav-1 are of paramount interest in oncology because are up-regulated in many cancer cells. Moreover, Cav-1 is responsible for human albumin uptake and trafficking, which have been recently demonstrated to play a pivotal role in pancreatic tumor growth [10]. Notably, a very recent work has shown that caveolin-mediated endocytosis is critical in targeted chemotherapy. For instance, for the uptake of conjugates composed by human albumin and chemotherapeutics [11].

Actually, materials can be also internalized by cells by following active pathways independent by clathrin- and caveolae-endocytosis. These routes rely on cholesterol and have been classified, according to GTPase role in the endocytic mechanisms, to Arf6-, Cdc42- and Rhoa- dependent endocytosis.

However, the relative lack of literature on this topic reflects the poor understanding of the process and of the intracellular late stage of the internalized materials [12].

The accurate knowledge of endocytic mechanisms is of critical importance in the development of nanotheranostics because: i) nanomaterials can be decorated with ligands that bind specific receptor for active cellular targeting, and ii) the intracellular fate of the internalized nanomaterials is closely related to the uptake pathway. For instance, the clathrin-coated vesicles turn into early endosomes following depolymerization of the coating and the internal pH drop to 5.9–6 upon maturation in late endosomes, and to 5 when they become lysosomes [13]. Also macropinosomes undergo a similar fate in the late stages. Alternatively, in non-phagocytic cells, macropinosomes mature independently from lysosomal pathway and, eventually, fuse again with plasma membrane returning most of the internalized material back to extracellular environment [14].

It is important to note that the strongly acidic environment in lysosomes is ascribed to the primary function of these organelles, that is the digestion of undesired internalized macromolecules. The environment inside lysosomes is able to partially or completely biodegrade many drugs drastically reducing their activity. Thus, drug carries should avoid this fate or provide lysosomal escape pathways.

On the other hand, caveolin-mediated endocytosis seems to produce vesicles able to avoid lysosomal degradation by fusing to cytoplasmic organelles. There are several ligands that promote internalization by caveolae, including many pathogens and viruses. For instance, investigations on the endocytic pathway of SV40 virus have demonstrated that caveolin-mediated internalization is triggered by specific ligands and lead to grape-like multicaveolar vesicles (called caveosomes) that have a neutral pH and do not fuse with lysosomes [15]. Nonetheless, some works have reported data supporting the hypothesis that caveolae vesicles can transiently fuse with conventionally endocytosed vesicles (*i.e.* early endosomes). Remarkably, the authors that have reported the first observations on caveosomes have also confirmed that caveolae actually followed the classical endocytic pathway until the formation of early endosomes. Thus, the vesicular bodies called caveosomes can be modified in late endosomes or lysosomes, and their formation can be due to the overexpression of Cav-1 [16].

Obviously, non-degradative internalization pathways such as caveolin-mediated endocytosis have generated increasing excitement as potential drug delivery mechanism to employ. For instance, Voigt and co-workers have reported caveolae targeting *in vitro*, simply through decoration of NPs with negatively-charged lipophilic moieties [17]. Exploiting the up-regulation of Cav-1 expression in endothelial cells, with respect to epithelial cells, they delivered lipid NPs coated with anionic polyelectrolites to cultured HUVEC and HeLa cells. They reported that, among polymers with similar electrical charge, the most lipophilic one (polystyrene sulfonate) have demonstrated the highest affinity for caveolin-mediated endocytosis. Thus, a specific cell targeting and selective cellular uptake mechanism were achieved simultaneously without the need for receptor-ligand targeting strategy.

Similarly, the employment of sphingolipids to decorate the surface of NPs has resulted to be effective to targeting caveolae; providing enhanced internalization in endothelial cancer cells. In particular, chemotherapeutic drug oxaliplatin was loaded into sphingolipids NPs micelles and the efficiency investigated on colorectal cancer. By exploiting overexpression of caveolae in neoplasms' cells with respect to healthy cells, a substantial specificity and enhanced therapeutic efficiency was achieved [18].

An alternative approach relies in escaping the lysosome ensuing the standard endocytosis uptake rather than employing non-lysosomal endocytic pathways. In 1997, Behr proposed an escaping mechanism based on the buffering capability of certain polycationic polymers [19]. In the so called "proton-sponge

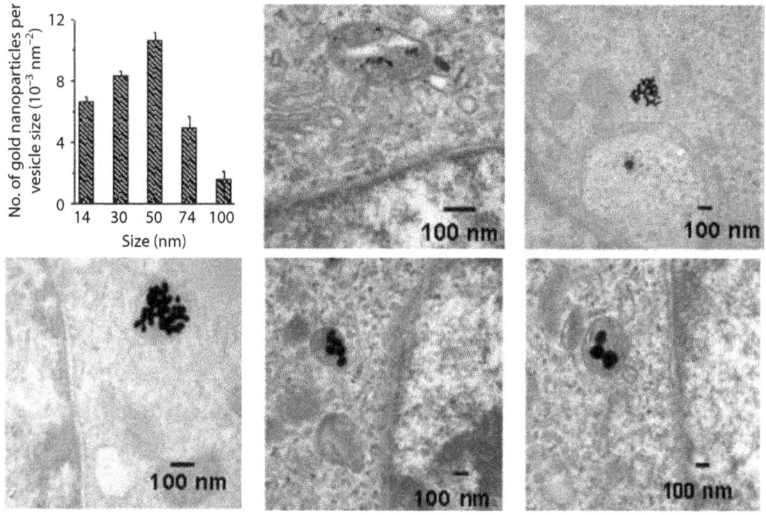

Figure 4.2 (Top) Cellular uptake histogram of gold NPs in the range 14–100 nm (left) and TEM images of the of 14 nm (center), 30 nm (right), 50 nm (bottom, left), 74 nm (bottom, center) and 100 nm (bottom, right) NPs trapped in vesicles in HeLa cells [33]. Reproduced with permission from [33]. Copyright 2006 American Chemical Society. Reproduced with permission from [32]. Copyright 2006 American Chemical Society

hypothesis", non-protonated amines of poly(ethylenimine) (PEI) absorb protons entering in the lysosomal compartment and lead to an increase in proton injection. The unbalanced ionic concentration inside the vesicle recalls an influx of water molecules and Cl^- ions, altering its the osmotic equilibrium and finally results in its swelling. This effect combined with the swelling of PEI due to the electrostatic repulsion between protonated amines, eventually cause the rupture of lysosomal membrane and the release of internalized material in the cytosol.

The findings of Behr *et al.* were the base for the development of several other materials able to provide the proton-sponge effect for lysosomal escape [20–24]. Some years after the report of Behr, Won *et al.* published an interesting perspective in which the fascinating proton-sponge theory was discussed from a critical point of view. The authors highlighted some untreated issues, including the poor knowledge on the chemical mechanisms at the basis of the proton buffering and the lack of evidence of the osmotic disruption of lysosomal membrane [25].

Other strategies to bypass lysosomal degradation involve the employment of moieties that mimic the endocytic uptake of some viruses. For instance, Chen *et al.* developed a synthetic polymer modified with a peptide sequence showing membrane-lytic ability [26]. Remarkably, the polymer is designed in order to change conformation in function of the environmental pH. The authors successfully exploited this virus-mimicking polymer for gene therapy. They have demonstrated a cytoplasm DNA release orders of magnitude higher than from controls employing the proton sponge effect of branched PEI.

An impressive amount of works has been published regarding the enhanced cellular uptake properties of cell penetrating peptides (CPPs). The success of CPPs is due to their endosomal escape capability. The first CPP was inspired by the basic domain of the Trans-Activator of Transcription protein (Tat) of the Human Immunodeficiency Virus (HIV), which was found to promote spontaneous cellular uptake of the virus [27]. However, the original Tat peptide sequence induces cellular uptake through all possible endocytic pathways, suffering from vesicle entrapment. This challenge pushed many groups towards the engineering of modified Tat sequences that could provide vesicle escape while retaining their internalization properties [28–30]. On this regard, an interesting class of chimeric peptides with membrane-disruptive properties has been engineered by combining arginine-rich Tat motif with sequences from α-helical antimicrobial peptides Cecropin-A and Melittin [31]. *In vitro* tests have shown that this modular peptide combined an efficient translocation towards intracellular vesicles with cytoplasm localization ensuing endosomal membrane disruption while inducing no significant toxicity.

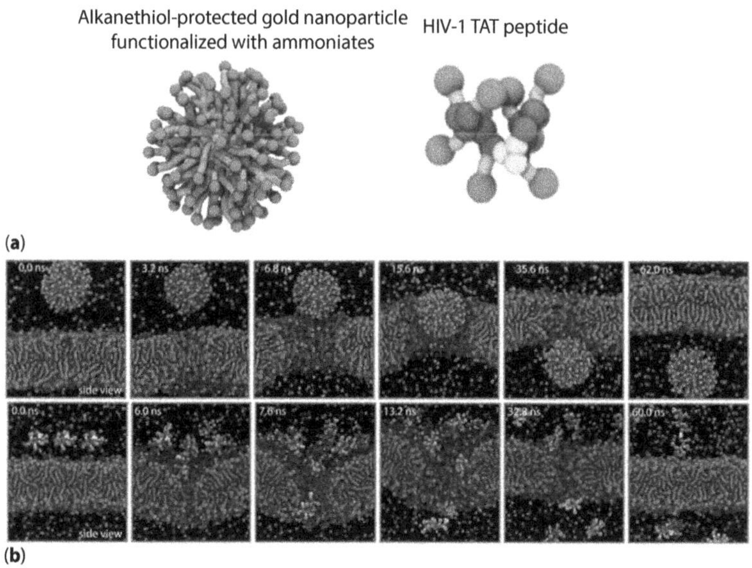

Figure 4.3 (a) Individual components employed for the simulation and (b) kinetics of spontaneous uptake for a cationic gold NP (top) and HIV-1 Tat peptide (bottom) [52]. Reprinted with permission from [52]. Copyright 2003 American Chemical Society. Reprinted with permission from [51]. Copyright 2003 American Chemical Society

4.1.2 Physio-Chemical Dependence of Nanomaterials Uptake

Physio-chemical properties of macromolecules, including size, shape, hydrophobicity and electric charge, are the result of an evolutionary adaptation reflecting their biological role. For instance, viruses have evolved in several shapes, such as icosahedral or rod-shaped, which dictated their specific cellular internalization and retention. The same argument applies to nanomaterials: the design of NPs should hence be guided by the final biological application [32].

As we briefly mentioned above for caveolae, size is one of the key parameter governing cellular internalization. Several studies reported that for spherical NPs, the optimal size for promoting internalization is 50 nm. For instance, Chithrani *et al.*, reported a systematical study on the cellular uptake of gold NPs in the range 14–100 nm on HeLa cells, providing qualitative evidences that the highest level of internalization occurs for NPs of 50 nm [33]. The same authors have also investigated the size-dependent uptake of gold NPs coated by transferrin, in order to study the clathrin-mediated endocytic pathway. The optimal size for NPs uptake was confirmed, and a linear relationship between NPs size and exocytosis was observed. Briefly, they have reported the highest excretion percentage for 14-nm diameter NPs in three different cell lines [34]. The authors have speculated that the rate of exocytosis is related to the ligand coverage on NPs.

A similar study was conducted by Zhu and co-workers. They have investigated the cellular uptake of silica NPs in the range 50–300 nm on HeLa cells. They observed that particle size affected both the amount of internalized particles and the endocytic route. While cellular uptake of the largest NPs occurred only through clathrin-mediated endocytosis, NPs around 170 nm were internalized also through caveolin dependent pathway [35]. Their work also confirmed the previous findings on gold NPs, *i.e.* the highest amount of internalized NPs occurred for particles whose diameter was around 50 nm [36]. Notably, similar results have been documented for the internalization of polystyrene and iron oxide NPs, whose maximum uptake was achieved for NPs of 30–50 nm of diameter [37, 38].

Overall, there is a widespread consensus about the optimal size for cellular uptake of spherical NPs. Another widely investigated factor affecting the rate of internalization of nanomaterials is their shape.

In this regard, several groups compared the cellular uptake of spherical NPs versus elongated ones, such as rods. Common findings are: i) elongated NPs are less internalized with respect to nanospheres, and ii) increasing the aspect ratio of rods dramatically decreases the cellular uptake. For instance, Arnida *et al.* reported *in vitro* an increase of macrophage uptake for spherical gold NPs with respect to nanorods through inductively-coupled plasma mass (ICP-MS) analyses [39]. Meng and co-workers provided a more detailed investigation upon the cellular response to slight variations in the aspect ratios of rod-like silica NPs [40]. The authors evaluated the rate and abundance of NPs uptake in two cancer cell lines, with particles whose aspect ratio varied in the range 1–4.5. Their results demonstrated that cells were able to discern slight differences in nanorods aspect ratio, and internalize at higher rate particles with an intermediate aspect ratio of 2.1–2.5. The authors also claimed that macropynocitosis is somehow responsible for this selective internalization.

A common inaccuracy of most of the earlier studies on the dependence of cellular uptake on the shape of nanomaterials relies on the comparison among NPs with non-comparable sizes or with different surface functionalization. Hence, it is not easy to highlight a net shape dependence whereas other physiochemical parameters are not fixed. To address this issue, Florez *et al.* synthesized prolate polymeric NPs with different aspect ratios by stretching spherical NPs, therefore keeping the same volume, composition and surface chemistry among all the samples [41]. Internalization of these NPs was investigated *in vitro* on both stem cells and cancer cell lines. Again, a substantial decrease in the internalization rate was found by increasing the aspect ratio of NPs independently from the cell type.

Based on these increasing experimental evidences many groups performed computational analyses to shed light on the altered internalization kinetics of anisotropic nanomaterials [42]. Molecular dynamics simulations on passive endocytosis have provided other evidences on the mechanisms through which elongated particles are internalized in cells respect to spherical NPs. In agreement with the experimental evidences, cellular uptake of high aspect ratio NPs is slowed by their orientation, which the authors termed *submarine mode*, with the long axis parallel to plasma membrane. This mode induced an incomplete membrane wrapping, leading to unstable endocytic states and hindering the uptake. On the other hand, endocytosis is favored for spherical NPs and for low aspect ratio rod-like NPs, whose long axis is perpendicular to the membrane during the uptake (*rocket mode*), fastening the internalization [43].

The most prominent feature driving the interaction between nanomaterials and biological entities is the surface coating. The surface coating of NPs has been finely engineered during the past decades in order to achieve optimal cellular uptake and non-degradative intracellular fate. In particular, surface electrical charge has been demonstrated to dramatically affect NPs access to the cytosol. Early studies documented an enhanced uptake of charged NPs by non-phagocytic cells with respect to the neutral counterpart [44]. In particular, cationic NPs are generally internalized more massively respect to negative charged NPs. This trend was confirmed for various nanomaterials, among which: liposomes, metal-based NPs including gold, silver and iron oxide, silica NPs and polymeric NPs such as polystyrene and chitosan [45–50]. Actually, it has been widely recognized that translocation of cationic nanomaterials across plasma membrane is highly effective since it occurs through its physical disruption. Indeed, electrostatic interactions with positively charged NPs, regardless of their shape, size or chemical composition, often lead to erosion, thinning or creation of holes inside the lipid bilayer [51].

This internalization route is known as direct translocation and is a non-endocytic energy-independent process allowing for fast and massive cellular uptake of nano-objects. These features tickled the interests of many researchers as a potential dodge for enhanced intracellular delivery. For instance, Lin and co-workers provided molecular dynamics simulations to evaluate and compare the uptake kinetics of cationic NPs and Tat peptides through a model cell membrane (Figure 4.3). They have observed that both NPs and Tat spontaneously translocate the membrane with extremely similar kinetics, and form transient nanosized pores [52]. Interestingly, they reported that the spontaneous uptake of cationic NPs is related to the transmembrane potential, which is lowered at each pore creation owing to the increase in intracellular Ca^{2+} concentration. After reaching a certain number of membrane pores, the transmembrane potential is depleted and particles are internalized through standard endocytic pathways, with a slower kinetic, until the potential is restored.

4.1.3 Cytotoxicity

Once in cells, a prominent aspect regarding nanomaterials is the biological response to NPs uptake. Toxicity assessments are firstly performed *in vitro*, as easier to control, less time-consuming and cheaper than in vertebrate or *in vivo* tests. Moreover, for ethical reasons, it is highly recommended to perform exhaustive computational and *in vitro* screenings previous to animal testing.

The very first test able to provide preliminary information about the toxicity of a nanomaterial is the optical bright-field microscopy inspection of cells in order to assess alterations in morphology. Indeed, visual inspection is somewhat predictive of materials toxicity, as factors including proliferation, spreading and rounding are closely related to cells viability. For instance, Bhatia and co-workers reported a high degree of correlation between visual inspection and quantitative cytotoxicity assays on 3T3 fibroblasts cell culture interacting with nanomaterials [53]. In another work, electron microscopy inspection of cells morphology has been taken as reliable parameter to evaluate the toxicity of carbon based nanomaterials on cultured human macrophages [54].

More quantitative viability assays usually involve the employment of colorimetric tests that exploit either loss of plasma membrane integrity or organelles activity in order to assess the number of live/dead cells through dyes quantification. One of the most widely used viability assay is the trypan blue exclusion test, which relies on the permeation of a dye in the cytosol through damaged plasma membranes. Optical observations allow distinguishing between dead cells which are stained in blue, and live ones, that appear colorless. Several groups have evaluated the biocompatibility of sundry nanomaterials by monitoring their cytotoxicity by this assay, or through permeation in the cytoplasm of other moieties such as Neutral Red and propidium iodide [55, 56]. A more complex and accurate colorimetric assay for simultaneous detection of live and dead cells involves the use of two chemicals, *i.e.* calcein acetoxymethyl (AM) and ethidium homodimer. Calcein AM is converted in its green fluorescent form after diffusing into the cytosol by the action of intracellular esterases, while red fluorescent ethidium homodimer stains damaged or dead cells, as a membrane-impermeable molecule [57].

Other colorimetric tests are employed to evaluate cytotoxicity by the quantification of organelles metabolic activity. For instance, vital cells are characterized by an intense mitochondrial dehydrogenase activity, which can be assessed by employing tetrazolium salts. This chemical is reduced by mitochondrial enzymes producing formazan dyes, whose absorbance intensity reflects cell viability. One of the most employed salt for this assay is the 3-(4,5-dimethylthia-zol-2-yl)-2,5-diphenyl tetrazolium bromide (MTT), which is a pale-yellow salt which is reduced to a water insoluble blue dye inside live cells. MTT assay has been exploited to evaluate the *in vitro* cytotoxicity of many kinds of nanomaterials, including carbon-based, gold NPs, iron oxide NPs, quantum dots, and lipid-based NPs [58–67]. Unfortunately, MTT suffers from some drawbacks, such as the extremely poor water solubility. This implies the addition of organic solvents, such as dimethyl sulfoxide (DMSO), to solubilize the dye. Furthermore, MTT-formazan insoluble crystals are needle-shaped, and their precipitation could be cytotoxic itself, invalidating the assay. Some of these disadvantages have been overcome by the implementation of water soluble tetrazolium salts (WSTs), which showed lower cytotoxicity and no need for organic solvents to be solubilized, while maintaining the same operating principle of other tetrazolium salts based assays [68].

Remarkably, several reports indicate that colorimetric tests must be handled with care before drawing conclusions about the degree of toxicity of nanomaterials, since many of them can interfere with the assays [69]. For example, formazan is a strongly lipophilic compound that has been demonstrated to be stored in the intracellular space according to the availability of lipids. This has to be taken into account when performing MTT assays with liposomes, since an increase of intracellular NPs-derived lipids could bring to an anomalous accumulation of formazan in the cytosol, strongly interfering with the outcome of the assay [70]. Another issue is related to the interference of light scattering from NPs with the absorbance measurements during colorimetric assays. Indeed, both MTT and WSTs assays rely on absorbance measurements in a range of wavelengths that can match the absorbance maxima of some plasmonic NPs, hence producing misleading results. Many efforts to reduce the interference of plasmonic NPs with the optical readout of these assays have reduced but not completely solved false-positive or false-negative results. Some strategies include a preliminary quantification of NPs absorbance to be subtracted for a differential measurement, and the inclusion of a centrifugation step to remove NPs prior to viability assay [71]. Yet, metal NPs introduce other sources of interference apart from spectral superposition of the absorbance peaks. For instance, it was reported that silver and iron oxide NPs can either induce the reduction of MTT- and WSTs-formazan, hence producing an apparent increase in cell viability, or bind the dyes shifting their absorption peak, resulting in an artifact reduction of the viability [72]. Similar results were found for TiO_2 NPs, which stimulated tetrazolium reduction in the extracellular environment, producing false viability results [73].

Notably, other sources of interference with colorimetric assays were observed for non-plasmonic NPs through different pathways. Fisichella and co-workers have reported that toxicity assessment of silica NPs with MTT assay produced an overestimation of NPs toxicity, owing to the peculiar interaction of those particles with formazan, whose exocytosis was accelerated in HeLa cells line and astrocytes [74]. The authors claimed that a possible explanation for this behavior could be the interaction of NPs with intracellular vesicle trafficking, including formazan-loaded vesicles. The authors also suggest that this result may be not peculiar of silica NPs, whereas it may occur with any other type of nanomaterials. Hence, it is recommended that a crosscheck with multiple assays should be performed when evaluating nanomaterials toxicity, in order to produce reliable results.

The aforementioned assays correlate cytotoxicity to plasma membrane integrity or organelles activity, providing a fast and inexpensive tool for quantitative evaluation of live and death cells. Even though no information is given regarding the mechanisms that led to cell death. Other *in vitro* assessment techniques are required to shed light on the mechanisms that led to cell toxicity. Several tests have been designed, for instance, to assess if nanomaterials produce genotoxicity (*i.e.* damages to nucleic acids). Most of them are still colorimetric tests employing DNA-intercalating dyes, such as propidium iodide, to quantify the amount of damaged DNA ensuing exposure to NPs. One example is the comet assay, which is basically a gel electrophoresis in which dye-tagged intact DNA is displayed in the head of the electrophoretic run, whilst damaged DNA pieces migrate away in the tail of the run, depicting a comet. The amount of dye in the comet is then quantified to evaluate the genotoxicity of the nanomaterial. Several groups have reported the use of this assay to investigate the safety of silver NPs towards plants, murine and human cultured cells including epithelial cells, stem cells, blood cells, fibroblasts and cancer cells [75–80]. The general outcome of these tests is: silver NPs induce acute genotoxicity causing DNA strand break and purine base damage, often related to oxidative stress following the production of ROS. Similar results were observed on many metal oxide NPs, such as titanium, zinc and bismuth oxide NPs [81–84].

On the other hand, many nanomaterials can be considered safe with respect to DNA damage. In particular, Barnes *et al.* employed comet assay on rat fibroblasts exposed to different amounts of silica NPs, reporting no significant NPs-induced genotoxicity. Notably, the authors performed the experiments independently in two separate laboratories with the same outcome, confirming the robustness and reproducibility of the assay [85]. For a comprehensive review regarding the genotoxic effects of a number of nanomaterials, the readers are referred to the work of Magdolenova and co-workers [86]. Notably, the authors also highlighted many factors affecting the genotoxic response, including the physiochemical properties of nanomaterials and the experimental conditions [87].

4.2 Body Level (*in vivo*)

In the previous section, we have treated the biological interaction of nanomaterials at the cellular level, highlighting cellular uptake pathways, intracellular fate and cytotoxicity. From an experimental point of view, those investigations forego the studies on the interactions between nanomaterials and a whole organism, as already discussed above. Nevertheless, from a medical perspective, the cellular level is the final stage in the development of nanotheranostics from the bench to clinics. Indeed, as for any drugs, nanotheranostics can be administered at body level through a number of routes including oral administration, inhalation, intravenous injection, and transdermal application [87]. After administration, nanomaterials encounter a series of hurdles in their path towards the target for which they have been designed, which are described in this section.

4.2.1 Blood Circulation

Opsonization

After direct injection in the bloodstream, nanomaterials are in a complex biological environment rich of blood constituent (*e.g.* red and white blood cells and platelets) and proteins that are likely to interact with them. Hence, one of the very first barriers faced by nanomaterials is the opsonization, *i.e.* the surface coverage by proteins called opsonins, which dramatically

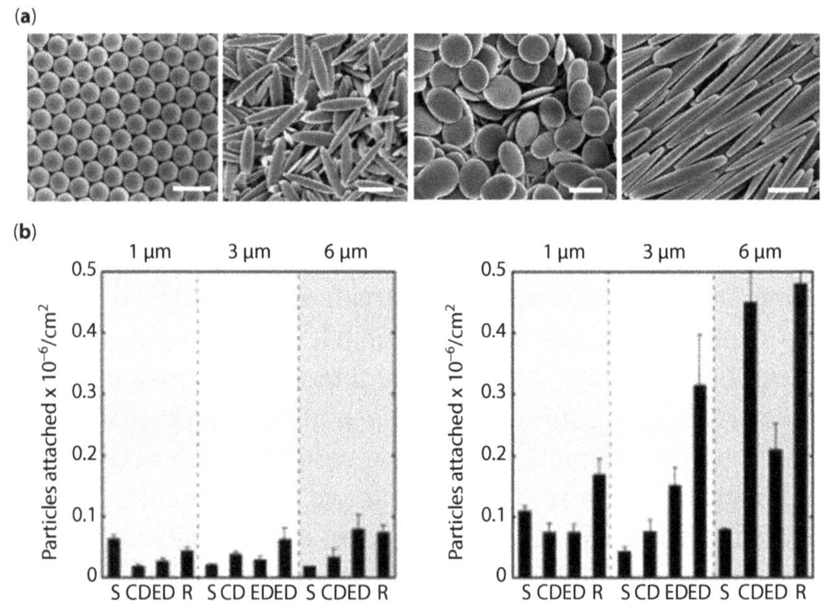

Figure 4.4 (a) SEM images of particles tested for vasculature adhesion assessment and (b) results of adhesion assay (S = spheres, ED = elliptical disks, CD = circular disk, R = rods) [124]. Adapted from [124] with permission of Elsevier

increase their elimination by macrophages. The formation of a thick protein corona around the particles often frustrates the efforts aimed at developing a stabilizing layer at a bench level, also inhibiting targeting moieties. On this regard, proteins that tightly bind to NPs and display a slow desorption kinetic contribute to the so called hard corona, whereas macromolecules that interact with the first layer of adsorbed proteins form the soft corona. Since each nanomaterial bears a certain affinity to different functional groups, it is hard to declare if a protein will contribute to the creation of soft or hard corona. Nevertheless, the study published by Aggarwal and co-workers report that there is some proteins, including fibrinogen, albumin and immunoglobulin, that are ubiquitous in the corona of all tested NPs [88].

The exact mechanisms at the basis of protein coverage of nanomaterials is still not completely elucidated, while a number of interactions are believed to drive their adsorption, including chemical affinity towards cysteine residues or entropy-driven binding. However, it has been largely recognized that opsonization is deeply related to the physiochemical features of nanomaterials. For instance, Piella and co-workers have recently reported that citrate-stabilized spherical gold NPs interact in different manners with proteins according to their size. The authors exposed NPs with diameters ranging from 3.5 to 150 nm to serum-containing cell culture media, identifying some threshold sizes which marked different regimes of protein corona formation. NPs smaller than 12 nm were partially coated by an incomplete layer of proteins, whereas particles from 12 to 80 nm displayed a dense protein monolayer, indicative of a full corona. Finally, in bigger NPs (>80 nm), the citrate coating was shielded by a thick corona made up by of two or three protein layers, behaving similarly to flat surfaces [89]. This result was confirmed by findings from similar investigations on polymer and silica nanospheres, in which protein corona formation is affected by particles size [90–92]. In general, the evidence that smaller spherical NPs are less prone to protein binding has been addressed to the increase in surface curvature.

Surface charge is another factor that critically contributes to the modulation of the protein corona. Several indications suggest that highly charged NPs, either positive or negative, show an accelerated corona formation kinetic with respect to neutral ones [93]. Some investigations on positively charged NPs have reported that they suffer from rapid clearance from the bloodstream owing to immediate binding by opsonins and macrophage sequestration. Concurrently, also negatively charged NPs suffer protein corona formation that lowering their zeta potential compromising their native stability [94]. On the other hand, neutral NPs are intrinsically poor stable as lacking of electrostatic stabilization, hence other approaches have been investigated to limit protein adsorption while increasing colloidal stability.

One of the most widely diffused antifouling coating to confer stealth ability to nanomaterials over opsonization is PEG polymer, which have been extensively adopted [95–99]. For example, Stolnik *et al.* demonstrated that PLGA NPs undergo drastic reduction of serum albumin adsorption, when coated with PEG-PLA copolymers [100]. Even the first FDA-approved nanodrug, Doxil®, owes part of his success to the stealth feature imparted by PEG coating [101]. The antifouling capability towards opsonins adhesion was addressed to the steric hindrance of the water layer formed by PEG coating. However, the extensive use of PEG coating has brought to several drawbacks that have motivated the investigation of novel approaches to evade macrophage clearance. One issue is related to the pharmacokinetics of repeated injection of PEGylated nanomaterials, which cause the so called accelerated blood clearance. It was firstly reported by Dams and co-worker that repeated weekly injections of PEG-stabilized liposomes. They have observed a dramatic decrease of blood circulation half-life of liposomes in rats and rhesus monkeys, with a parallel increase in the sequestration rate by macrophages [102]. It is generally accepted that this phenomenon arise since the first injection of PEG elicits an immune response that produce anti-PEG antibodies, in particular immunoglobulin-M, that accelerated blood clearance of the following injections [103]. Another issue is related to the steric hindrance formed by the aqueous layer around PEG coating which, despite promoting camouflage against macrophage clearance, results in poor interaction with target cell membrane thereby lowering both cellular uptake and eventually lysosomal escape [104, 105].

Since these concerns have hampered the medical translation of PEGylated nanocarriers, a number of PEG-free approaches for affording prolonged blood circulation have been proposed. For instance, other polymeric coatings have been explored, including poly(amino acids), polyglycerols and polysaccharides [106]. An interesting alternative was proposed by Sawant and co-workers, who combined the stealth capability of PEG with and endogenous-triggered targeting ability. They proposed a pH sensitive moiety composed by PEG and a cleavable linker which shield the carriers at pH range 7.4–8.0, and is detached from the particle at slightly acidic environments, as in tumor environment [107]. Another valid alternative to PEG was identified in zwitterionic molecules such as polybetaines, which combined anti-opsonization properties with the availability of multiple functional groups. These moieties have been exploited to modify a number of nanomaterials, including iron oxide, silica, PLGA and gold NPs. Ranalli *et al.* have recently reported the synthesis of biomimetic lipid vesicles that jointly combine the stealth behavior of zwitterionic lipopeptides with the targeting capability of transferrin-recognizing aptamers. These vesicles were benchmarked against plain liposomes and PEG-decorated liposomes with respect to protein adsorption rate in serum, yielding excellent antifouling ability and unaltered targeting effectiveness towards cancer cells [108].

Interestingly, many groups proposed biomimetic approaches to produce cell-like carriers that are able to be not identified by the immune system as foreign guests. This approach includes loading of naturally occurring exosomes or functionalizing synthetic nanomaterials, such as silica NPs, with a coating obtained from purified cellular membranes (*e.g.* leukocytes) [109, 110].

Hematologic Disorders

Another concern regarding the use of nanomaterials *in vivo* is their interaction with blood components, which could produce hematologic disorders such as hemolysis and thrombosis. Although there is not a unique hemolytic disease and each one has its related symptoms, most of them are characterized by an increase in free hemoglobin in the blood [111]. Nanomaterials may interact with red blood cells within the vascular compartment by damaging their plasma membrane, resulting in an increase of extracellular levels of free hemoglobin. Once in the bloodstream, free hemoglobin is rapidly bound by haptoglobin protein, which exposes the complex to macrophage clearance, hence inducing hemoglobin depletion. A number of nanomaterials have been demonstrated to induce red blood cells hemolysis, among which silica NPs, dendrimers, titanium oxide NPs, silver NPs and carbon fullerenes [112–116]. This severe issue hampers the use of engineered nanomaterials, as they would produce severe diseases immediately after systemic injection and even before their theranostic action is accomplished. Some groups have reported the synthesis of either bare nanomaterials or properly functionalized ones that do not display any hemolytic activity. For instance, Fornaguera *et al.* have investigated the interactions of PLGA NPs with blood components, reporting alteration in blood coagulation only for high concentrations of injected NPs. Noteworthy, they did not observed hemolytic activity towards erythrocytes regardless of surface functionalization of PLGA NPs [117].

On the other hand, a proper surface functionalization can deeply reduce the hemolytic activity and the toxicity of NPs. Yildirim and co-workers reported that the significant hemolytic activity of silica NPs can be related to the abundance of silanol groups exposed on their surface. Indeed, the significant hemolysis produced by bare silica NPs can be reduced by their functionalization with organosilane monomers [118]. Similarly, a marked decrease in NPs-induced hemolysis was reported for PEG-coated gold NPs, if compared to freshly synthesized NPs stabilized by their mother surfactant [119]. Interestingly, Saha *et al.* demonstrated that exploiting protein corona is a smart approach to mitigate the hemolytic effect of gold NPs. They synthesized nine sets of gold NPs which were chemically functionalized in order to bear increasing degree of hydrophobicity. All the particles showed significant toxicity towards red blood cells which was more pronounced by increasing hydrophobicity. Nevertheless, when the NPs were incubated in serum prior to the assessment, a significant decrease of hemolysis was observed even after 24 h incubation with erythrocytes [119].

Blood Circulation and Extravasation

Another important argument related to blood circulation is the hydrodynamic behavior of nanomaterials when flowing into the blood vessels. Indeed, after injection, nanomaterials should flow easily through the capillaries and they have to escape the blood flow and extravasate to reach the target sites. Many groups have investigated intravascular transport of nanomaterials either through theoretical models or experimentally by means of microfluidics devices [121–123]. It is well recognized that in order to evade the vasculature, NPs have to drift from the blood flow streamlines and flow near the capillary walls to escape the circulation. In order to promote extravasation, nanomaterials can be engineered by learning from naturally blood-occurring particles, as platelets, that drift from the blood flow to locate damaged vessel walls (a phenomenon called margination).

On this regard, Gentile and co-workers reported a comparative study on margination ability of silica discoidal particles against spherical and quasi-hemispherical ones using a microfluidic chamber. The margination was quantified as number of sedimented particles in the capillary in a selected ROI. The experiment outcome displayed a net increase in margination propensity for discoidal particles compared to the other two shapes [124]. Similar findings were obtained on polystyrene microparticles with various geometries. Their adhesion propensity was found to be higher for flattened particles compared to spherical ones, with the highest adhesion displayed by elongated particles (Figure 4.4) [125]. However, particles employed in these works are in the micrometer range, being well representative of the hydrodynamic behavior of blood cell components, whereas not suitable for simulating NPs motion in the blood flow.

On the other hand, a very recent work from Tang *et al.*, have demonstrated that also the density of nanomaterials plays a pivotal role in extravasation. By employing a class of ultrasmall metal NPs with the same size and surface chemistry but different densities, they have observed that passive tumor accumulation – thus extravasation – linearly decreased by decreasing the particle density [127]. Tan *et al.* reported a study based on a computational model for NPs circulation in a mimetic branched blood vessel, assessing the vessel adhesion ability of nanospheres against nanorods of different sizes and aspect ratios. The motion of 100 nm and 200 nm NPs is evaluated at single particle level, resulting in: i) increased vessel adhesion for smaller particles owing to higher diffusion, ii) orientation-dependent and adhesion of nanorods due to the varying contact area with the vessels and iii) higher vessels binding for nanorods with respect to nanospheres, whereas no direct correlation to their aspect ratio was found. Moreover, it was predicted that in a complex vasculature NPs display the highest binding rate with vessels in the branched regions [128]. This behavior plays a role of paramount importance when considered by the point of view of oncologists. Indeed, tumor growth and proliferation is strictly dependent to a concurrent accelerated angiogenesis which gives rise to a complex neovasculature greatly different from the one of healthy tissues. Capillaries within the tumors form a dense network of irregularly shaped vessels writhing and dilating with increasing tortuosity as the tumor matures. Hence, preferential adhesion of nanomaterials on branched regions of blood vessels would favor the interactions with those tissues, such as cancerous ones, which display an intricate branchy vasculature [129]. Moreover, several evidences have led to a general consensus on the enhanced leakiness of tumor vasculature with respect to normal one.

Blood vessels are composed mainly by endothelial cells which have one side facing the bloodstream and the other resting on basement membrane. There are different types of vessels, each one providing important physiological functions. The so-called continuous vessels are made by strictly packed endothelial cells slightly separated by tight gaps of less than 1 nm to a maximum of 5 nm. These gaps allow for extravasation of solutes and small molecules from the blood to the tissue, while impeding the leakage of large macromolecules. On the other hand, large molecules can diffuse from blood to the tissues when flowing in the fenestrated vessels. For instance, proteins can extravasate through these pores, called *fenestrae*, in the endothelium (whose diameter in physiological conditions lies in the range 5–12 nm) [130]. Moreover, early investigations on the leakage of NPs from blood capillaries have led to the formulation of the dual pore theory, according to which vessels are also endowed with an another class of pores with a diameter from 24 to 60 nm [131]. It is important to note that these pores are a separate concept from the discontinuous (or sinusoidal) vessels, whose pores are in the micrometer range thanks to a discontinuous basal lamina, which are located in those tissues where a fast diffusion of cells or materials is needed.

This picture is representative of normal tissue vasculature, though it is somehow misleading when considering neoplasms environment. Indeed, the endothelium of tumor blood vessels is anatomically defective and that cells are poorly aligned and their packaging is not so tight, hence larger fenestration are present. Also, basement membrane is frequently abnormal or even absent [132]. Furthermore, it is known from early reports that the blood flow in the tumor vessels is slow and that the leakage of large macromolecules through the vasculature is promoted also through the secretion of a permeability-enhancing factor. On the other hand, the retention of small molecules in tumor tissues is somehow inhibited by the hypervascularization of the area. In addition, tumors often lacks lymphatic drainage, thereby large molecules are retained for a long time [133]. Considered together, these phenomena have aroused enormous interests among oncologists, as the capability of tumors of retaining large objects, as nanomaterials, at a higher extent with respect to healthy tissues, results as a passive targeting route for selective delivery of chemotherapeutics. Termed enhanced permeability and retention effect (EPR), it has been the most underlying concept in the engineering of drug carriers for decades, holding the promise of simple and effective passive tumor targeting.

The first proof of the effectiveness of EPR *in vivo* was reported by Maeda, who employed dyes conjugated to a number of proteins of various molecular weights to visualize accumulation in tumor [134]. Based on that report, many drugs formulation were proposed until the first EPR-based polymeric formulation of a chemotherapeutic, named SMANCS, was clinically approved in Japan for the treatment of metastatic liver cancer [133]. Following this important result, other groups designed polymeric conjugates of chemotherapeutics claiming for the importance of EPR-driven tumor specific accumulation. For instance, *N*-(2-hydroxypropyl)methacrylamide (HPMA) copolymer has been extensively exploited for enhancing passive drug accumulation in cancer tissues. Many of these conjugates are still under investigation in clinical trials against a number

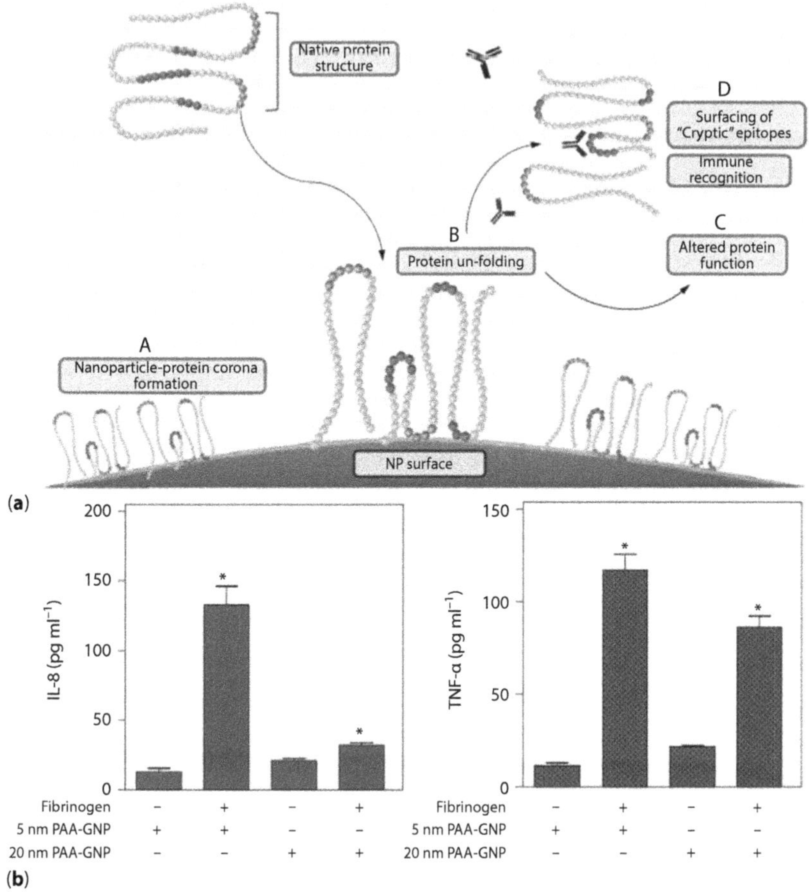

Figure 4.5 (a) Schematic depiction of the immune system recognition of hidden epitopes that become exposed following protein corona formation.
(b) interleukins (left) and tumor necrosis factors (right) secretion by THP-1 cells following exposure to fibrinogen and gold NPs of 5 and 20 nm [162, 163].
(a) reproduced with permission from [162]. (b) Reproduced with permission from [163]. Copyright 2010 Springer Nature.

of cancer models [135]. Also micellar encapsulation served as efficient route for enhancing the passive tumor accumulation through EPR. Polymeric micelles of 30 nm loaded by cisplatin, were shown to afford prolonged blood retention and specific accumulation at tumor site compared to the bare drug. Toxicity studies on these nanomicelles on mice and rats models also demonstrated that EPR significantly contributed to reduce the typical adverse effects following off-target deposition of cisplatin, including neurotoxicity and nephrotoxicity [136].

As most of the drug carriers proposed in the last decades have been engineered on the rationale of EPR effect, evidences have emerged that this effect is anything but a general concept applicable to all nanomaterials. EPR validity should be assessed on a case-by-case basis, as it produces the desired effect only when a complete set of conditions is jointly satisfied. First of all, size play a critical role in the efficacy of EPR effect, as NPs should be bigger than 10 nm to avoid extravasation through healthy vasculature and smaller than 100 nm to overcome specific macrophage clearance. Secondly, tumor environment should be devoid of lymphatic drainage to prevent clearance. However, only few case studies have reported the absence of lymph vessels in specific cancers, whereas the majority of solid tumors display an altered drainage located mostly in the periphery [137]. Moreover, fenestration in the vasculature itself should be sufficient to allow transfer of nanomaterials from the vessels to the tissue, meaning that no hurdles should be present between the vessel pore and the tissue.

Nevertheless, the chaotic biological environment of tumors does not refer exclusively to the intricate vasculature, as beyond the vessels, a complex cellular architecture could hamper the penetration of the particles that have escaped the bloodstream. Indeed, the presence of perycites, smooth muscle cells or fibroblast often act as a barrier against the filtration of extravasated material [140]. Furthermore, not all the tumors have fenestrated vessels, and even within a single tumor there is an enormous variability in the vasculature permeability, hence in some spots even the diffusion of material of 2–3 nm is hampered. Another issue related to the chaotic growth of tumors is that sometimes cancers have a low amount of capillaries sprinkling throughout the tissue, or the majority of the cells are far from the vasculature. This, apart from leading to the appearance of hypoxic regions which are the cause of resistance to numerous anticancer treatments, decreases the likelihood that nanomaterials reach the malignancy [141]. Finally, the contorted and leaky tumor vasculature poses some limitations to EPR, as the extravasation of plasma proteins and other macromolecules out of blood compartment often leads to an increased interstitial fluid pressure (IFP). Since the surrounding healthy tissues have a normal IFP, this unbalanced pressure induces nanomaterials to flow from the center of the tumor to the periphery, reducing the target retention [139].

Another concern on the effectiveness of EPR effect as tumor targeting strategy is related to the pathophysiological heterogeneity between tumors and the enormous differences that emerge when cancers are compared between human patients and murine models. Indeed, several investigations suggest that the peculiar angiogenesis in the tumor environment is dictated by the overexpression of a protein named vascular endothelial growth factor (VEGF). The up-regulation of VEGF and other growth factors that bind to tumor vasculature to promote angiogenesis are crucial for the exponential growth of the tumor mass in the first stage, until it reaches a pathological size (1–2 mm in mice). However, this abnormal secretion of VEGF, beside accelerating tumor growth, is one of the main reasons for the development of leaky and disordered vasculature, one of the key-points for the reliability of EPR effect [142]. Two important points have to be highlighted on this regard: i) not all the solid tumors display the same rate of VEGF production and, subsequently, the same disordered and damaged vasculature and ii) tumor progression rate in rodents model have an extremely accelerated kinetics if compared to humans, hence the angiogenesis is not directly comparable [143, 144].

Very recently, a comparative study concerning the heterogeneous efficacy of the EPR effect on 17 clinical studies was reported. Natfji and co-workers reported that the magnitude of nanomedicine retention is strictly correlated to tumor size and type. In particular, pancreatic, colon, stomach and breast cancer displayed the highest levels of accumulation, whereas the comparison between solid tumors of varying size was conducted by categorizing tumors into three classes according to their volume and progression stage: medium, large and very large [145]. The analyses showed that, while large tumors displayed the highest level of accumulation, only in 53% of the cases there was evidence of EPR effect. Conversely, medium ones retained a lower amount of nanomedicines, yet in 100% of the case studies there was a clear manifestation of EPR. This point is of paramount importance in understanding why EPR effect is often overrated when benchmarking animal models with human clinical studies. On one hand, clinically relevant solid tumors in mice have typically a size over 5 mm, reaching about 3% of mouse body weight. This, translated to humans, would be equivalent to a tumor mass of few kilograms, which is not a suitable condition for nanomedicine anticancer treatment [144]. On the other hand, most of the clinical studies on nanomedicines are performed on patients in an advanced disease state, hence there is a generalized lack of assessment on the performance of EPR in early stage cancers, both in animal models and clinical studies.

All these biological hurdles, together with the substantial decrease in passive targeting efficacy when translating from animal models to humans, have aroused disillusionment towards EPR effect. Plenty of reviews have been published in which EPR was evaluated from a critical point of view; sometimes the scenario is that nanomedicine should be reconsidered without considering EPR [141]. Nevertheless, some groups have dedicated efforts to enhance the passive targeting capability provided by EPR by, for instance, altering tumor blood flow either by administering vasoconstrictors or vasodilators. Another proposed strategy was to increase the permeability of tumor vasculature by opening tight junctions in the vascular endothelium by means of ultrasound-triggered cavitation [146]. A controversial solution is the administration of VEGF which, on one hand promotes the growth of disordered and leaky vasculature useful to enhance extravasation of nanomedicines, whereas on the other it could bring to undesirable growth of the tumor itself [147]. Alternatively, an opposite strategy consists in reducing the vascular leakage, either by administering VEGF inhibitors or anti-angiogenic drugs that reestablish vessels integrity, in order to reduce the interstitial fluid pressure that opposes to intra-tumor drug diffusion [148, 149]. Other promising strategies to enhance the EPR effect involve the co-delivery of nanomedicines jointly with photothermal, photodynamic and radiation therapy, and more complex routes which rely on the physical disruption of vessels and altering the tumor microenvironment to decrease its biological barriers. Most of these strategies are briefly summarized in a recent work published by Nakamura and co-workers, to which we refer the readers for further details [146].

4.2.2 Immune/Inflammatory Response

Regardless of the EPR effect, it is important to take into account that accumulation of nanomaterials in tumors rarely exceeds 5% of the administered dose. This percentage could be increased by proper functionalization of nanomaterials surface, either by means of active targeting moieties or through PEGylation, as previously discussed. The majority of the injected nanomaterials spread throughout the body for a certain amount of time, until being excreted or accumulated elsewhere in the organism. The details regarding the biodistribution of nanomaterials in the body will be discussed later, whereas now will be pointed out an important aspect related to the off-target distribution of nanomaterials: the immune system response. The immune system is a complex biological system that has the role of providing defense against foreign agents that are considered harmful for the organism. It is often divided in innate and adaptive immune system, where the first is highly reactive against any foreign intrusion and the latter is less responsive but provide memory of the intrusion in order to unleash an enhanced response in the subsequent encounter with the antigen. Almost all the direct adverse effects deriving from nanomaterials immunoactivation is driven by the innate immune system [150].

Basically, any foreign substance that is injected in the body is potentially considered an antigen, and the innate immune system react to its appearance by producing antibodies that block its spreading. It is straightforward to imagine that nanomaterials can be recognized as antigens, hence inducing an immune reaction in patients. One of the typical responses to the administration of nanomaterials is the immunostimulation, that is the production of immunoglobulins (antibodies). The most common immunostimulatory effects of nanomaterials are antigenicity and related adjuvant properties, immunosuppression, and inflammatory response [151].

Antigenicity is a rather rare effect directly resulting from nanomedicine. Indeed, it is based on the production of specific antibodies "anti-nanomaterial", though in most cases the antigenic immune response was induced by the decorative moieties rather than NPs themselves. Inflammation, instead, is a process in which the immune system elicits the production of signaling molecules known as cytokines to recruit other cells with the objective of removing a substance recognized as foreign. Early studies have been carried on regarding the antigenic properties of many NPs, including dendrimers and gold NPs, without revealing any antigenicity [152, 153]. However, recently, other findings suggested that PAMAM dendrimers induced toxicity in zebrafish embryos which was related to activation of the innate immune system, hence the immunomodulatory properties of nanomaterials in general should be reassessed [154]. In this context, Palomäki and co-workers explored the immunological effects of five different nanomaterials comprising TiO_2 NPs and silica coated TiO_2 NPs, ZnO NPs, single and multi-walled carbon nanotubes. The study was conducted *in vitro* on antigen bearing cells, finding that while ZnO NPs and the two TiO_2 NPs drastically stimulated immune response by the production of a number of interleukins, tumor necrosis factors and inflammation-related proteins, carbon nanotubes didn't produce any significant immunological response [155]. This result is surprising because other carbon-based nanomaterials were found to be immunostimulating. Indeed, C_{60} fullerenes were demonstrated to trigger the production of specific antibodies in mice. Notably, it was demonstrated that immunoglobulin response was directly induced by the nanomaterials, rather than their surface functional groups, hence the immune system provided a specific recognition pathway for fullerenes [156].

These disagreeing results could imply that immune responses may not be triggered solely by the chemical composition of the nanomaterials, yet a number of factors including size, shape and also the patient immunological anamnesis could play an important role in unleashing the immune response. Actually, there is no evidence that the immune system is able to recognize inorganic compounds as epitopes. Albeit some authors reported antibody affinity for certain materials such as magnetite and gallium arsenide, yet no evidences for the existence of specific antibodies against these materials have been reported [157]. There is only one group who reported the existence of human antibodies against specific nanomaterials, *i.e.* gold NPs [158]. Apart for this isolated report, chemical composition alone seems to be not enough to justify the immunomodulatory properties of some nanomaterials, thereby the triggering mechanism may originate from other properties.

On this regard, an interesting work published by Moyano *et al.*, attempted to shed light on the mechanisms at the basis of nanomaterials-triggered immunological responses by investigating the effect of surface hydrophobicity. They have tested immune activation elicited by gold NPs of fixed size and shape, modified with functional groups of increasing degree of hydrophobicity, towards splenocytes. Immune response was assessed as the level of expression of cytokines as a function of NPs hydrophobicity, reporting a linear correlation *in vitro*. This result is somehow expected, considering that hydrophobic molecules and proteins' parts are naturally present in the organism in a hidden form, as in physiological conditions they are shielded from the extracellular milieu. However, during cells necrosis, these molecules are exposed to interact with membrane specific receptor, eliciting an immune response. Nevertheless, the same experiments were carried out on mouse models, displaying again a linear increase of immune activation with increasing hydrophobicity, even though the highest hydrophobic NPs failed in inducing immune response. This result was reasonably ascribed by the authors to the complex behavior of nanomaterials *in vivo* ensuing systemic administration, whose biodistribution is severely altered in particular when their surface is highly hydrophobic [159].

It is important to note that immunomodulation is not necessarily an adverse effect leading to toxicity, yet it can be exploited for therapeutic purposes. Immune system, indeed, provide a system to protect the organism from foreign substances as well as against diseases hence, in principle, it can be stimulated for self healing. For instance, the mechanism through which vaccines protect the body from common diseases is the administration of agents that resemble specific disease-inducing pathogen in order to stimulate the immune cell to recognize it (memory effect). On this regard, several groups have started considering the possibility of exploiting the immune system in the struggle against cancer, either through the induction of inflammatory responses in the tumor microenvironment, or by targeting specific tumor antigens [160]. In this scenario, Chakraborty *et al.* have reported an investigation on the immunostimulatory properties of silver NPs for cancer therapy, assessing their ability of arresting the growth of a murine fibrosarcoma [161]. In this study, sarcoma was induced in mice chemically, by administering the carcinogenic 3-methylcholanthrene (3-MCA) and the tumor promoter phorbol myristate 13-acetate (PMA). The antigenic properties of Ag NPs were evaluated through a comparison among mice treated with carcinogenics only, and mice in which also Ag NPs coated with mouse serum albumin were injected. Tumor incidence, body weight and tumor size were monitored during 40 weeks, finding that mice treated with Ag NPs displayed: i) a significant delay in the appearance of the sarcoma (9 weeks), ii) no evidence of weight loss and iii) a shrinking in tumor size of more than half with respect to untreated mice. The authors claimed that anticancer activity was driven by immunostimulatory activity of Ag NPs as evidenced from the increase in the count of white blood cells, lymphocytes and granulocytes.

Attempting to give an explanation to this result, a straightforward speculation is that the immunomodulatory activity of NPs might be, in general, the result of protein corona formation. Indeed, it is reasonable that in a complex biological environment proteins are continuously modulating NPs corona, and several epitopes that are usually hidden become exposed once adsorbed on NPs surface [162]. For instance, Deng and co-workers reported that gold NPs interaction with plasma fibrinogen induces an immune response that ultimately leads to the release of inflammatory cytokines. Immunomodulatory response was ascribed to fibrinogen unfolding, that expose a binding site for macrophage recognition which is otherwise buried in the hydrophobic core of the protein [163]. This interpretation is based on the evidence that fibrinogen itself does promote interaction with macrophage receptor, and that immune system was stimulated only by NPs of a certain size. While 5 nm gold NPs promoted the secretion of cytokines such as intereleukins and tumor necrosis factors, fibrinogen adsorbed on 20 nm NPs produced a conformational change that hindered the access to the receptor binding site, thereby impairing cytokine production. The idea that nanomaterials acquire a new immunological identity once in the bloodstream, owing to corona formation, is relatively new. There are partial evidences that the immune system is somehow blind towards bare synthetic nanomaterials, whereby immunomodulation arising from opsonization follow different pathways. Notably, depending on the corona composition, immune activation was even shown to sustain either pro- or anti-tumoral activity [164].

4.2.3 Metabolism (RES, Degradation, Excretion and Persistence)

Reticuloendothelial System (RES)

Systemically administered nanomaterials are subject to several biophysical processes within the circulatory system that begin with opsonization and ultimately lead to rapid clearance from the bloodstream. Unluckily, in order to yield a convenient therapeutic action, nanomaterials should afford a sustained half-life in the blood flow and ultimately accumulate at target site. Nevertheless, as already discussed, innate immune system represents the body's first line of defense against the introduction of any foreign substance in the blood. In particular the blood is populated by macrophages, dendritic cells, and monocytes that recognize nanomaterials as antigens, thereby triggering an immune response that activate macrophages which promptly provide clearance from the circulatory system. These cells are part of the immune system and are referred to as reticuloendothelial system (RES). Following sequestration of the foreign substance in the blood, these cells accumulate in lymph nodes, lungs, liver and spleen, with the aim of metabolizing the foreign bodies.

Investigating the fate of nanomaterials *in vivo* is a topic of major interest in nanomedicine mainly for two reasons. First of all, in the perspective of drug delivery it is important to assess the amount of nanomaterials reaching the target and spreading throughout the body. Secondly, it is of paramount importance to know whether the off-target nanomaterials are retained in the body, in which site and how long. In a recent work published by Wilhelm and co-workers, the state of art of nanoparticle delivery to tumors is exhaustively reviewed. The authors performed a statistical analysis on the published papers regarding nanomedicine for cancer applications to assess the delivery efficiency of nanomaterials to tumors. The picture that came out is: a median of 0.7% of the injected dose of NPs reaches the tumor and this value not significantly varied in the last ten years [165]. It is legitimate to wonder what happens to the majority of injected nanomaterials that do not reach the target. On this regard literature provides plenty of works dealing with *in vivo* NPs pharmacokinetics, from which results that while biodistribution is dictated by their physiochemical properties, most of the nanomaterials share a common fate: accumulation in the RES.

For instance, tissue distribution of gold NPs of varying size was investigated by De Jong *et al.* in murine models. They analyzed organ uptake of spherical gold NPs in the broad size range 10–250 nm finding that particles bigger than 10 nm were found only in blood, liver and spleen, whereas 10 nm NPs were found also in kidneys, testis, lungs, heart and brain, with the highest percentage, again, in liver and spleen [166]. Similarly, Terentyuk and co-workers observed that PEGylated gold NPs of 15 nm were distributed almost equally in all the organs, while 50 nm NPs and 160 nm silica/gold nanoshells were accumulated in liver and spleen both in rats and rabbits (Figure 4.6a) [167]. In another study, PEG coated iron oxide NPs of 7.7 nm were doped with radioactive ^{111}In, whose decay was exploited for revealing their biodistribution in mice. After a transient concentration of NPs in the blood and in blood rich organs, including lungs, NPs accumulated stably in liver and spleen and their amount slowly decreased during 22 days owing to biodegradation or excretion (Figure 4.6c) [168]. Interestingly another group investigated the effect of shape in the biodistribution of silica NPs. In this work, spherical and rod-shaped silica NPs with varying aspect ratio were intravenously injected in mice and the organ distribution was evaluated. The study revealed that both spherical and rod NPs were mainly uptaken by liver and spleen, in particular with the longest rods that accumulated preferentially in the spleen [169]. This result was very recently confirmed by a similar work in which silica nanospheres and nanorods were administered orally to rats. Though long rods exhibited an enhanced residence time in the circulatory system, all the tested nanomaterials displayed the highest accumulation in the liver one week after administration (Figure 4.6b).

As immune activation of macrophages follows recognition pathways dictated by protein corona formation, it is not surprising that, regardless the chemical composition, the final fate of almost all the nanomaterials systemically administered is in the liver. Indeed, liver is the major metabolic regulator as well as one of the main organs assigned to immunosurveillance [171]. About 30% of total blood volume in the body flows every minute in the liver, thus it is straightforward to realize that it is the organ in which the greatest population of macrophages is retained. About 80–90% of all tissue macrophages in the body reside in the liver as Kupffer cells.

Liver contains the largest RES network in the body and has a particular anatomy that justifies its biological function and, at the same time, clarifies why nanomaterials accumulate there. When blood reaches the liver, its flow is considerably slowed by a capillary network shaped by the sinusoidal endothelial cells, in order to maximize the pathogens recognition by the immune system. These endothelial cells separate the bloodstream from

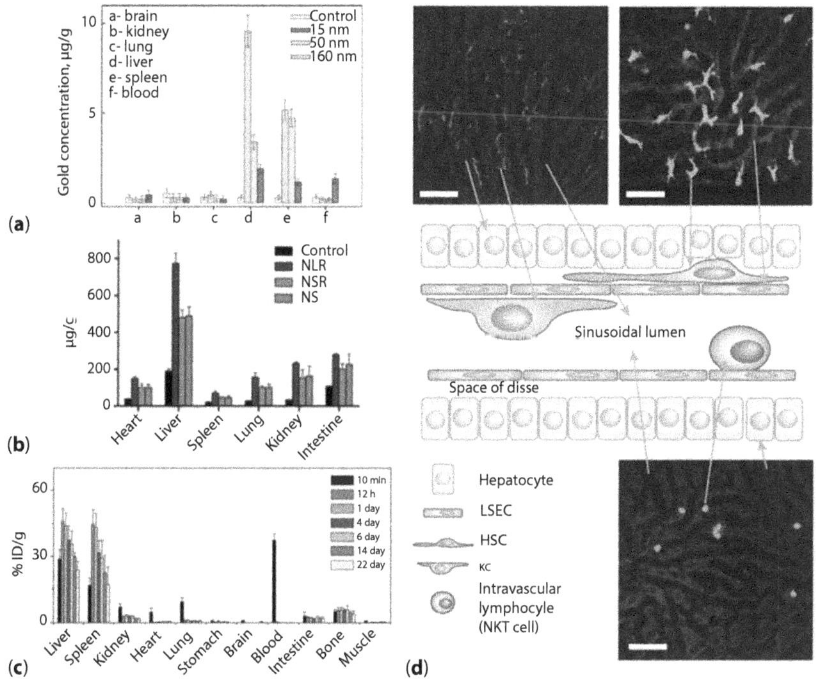

Figure 4.6 Biodistribution examples of nanomaterials with different chemical composition, size and shape in mice, including gold NPs (a), iron oxide NPs (b) and silica NPs (c), displaying preferential accumulation in the RES organs. Schematic depiction of a liver sinusoid in cross-section showing the main components in fluorescence microscopy images (d) [167, 168, 170, 171]. (a) Reproduced from [167] with permission of Elsevier. (b) Reproduced from [168] with permission of The Royal Society of Chemistry. (c) Reproduced with permission from [170]. Copyright 2017 Springer Nature. (d) Reproduced with permission from [171]. Copyright 2013 Springer Nature.

the hepatocytes, and the two are separated by a physical gap called space of Disse. Liver sinusoidal endothelial cells are not strictly packed, whereas they bear fenestration of 100–200 nm, which allows nanomaterials to cross into the space of Disse and get accumulated in the liver. It was suggested that, while nanomaterials are flowing in liver sinusoids, Kupffer cells engulf them through opsonin recognition and store the particles in order to metabolize them. Here, NPs undergo different fates depending on their chemical composition: organic NPs are degraded and eliminated in a reasonable amount of time while inorganic NPs, especially noble metal ones, cannot be degraded, resulting in their accumulation in the organ [165].

Similarly, to the liver, spleen is also sprinkled by a substantial blood flow, hence it is another important organ involved in the filtration of systemically injected nanomaterials. However, its importance in the metabolic activity towards nanotheranostics is often underestimated inasmuch as particles retention is considerably lower than in the liver. This is related to the considerably lower amount of blood that flows into the spleen, around 5% of the cardiac output [172]. However, it should be taken into account that spleen is considerably smaller than liver, thus it contribution to blood clearance is lower yet not negligible. The classically poorly considered role of spleen in pharmacokinetics has been very recently reconsidered from the perspective of nanomedicine [173]. Blood clearance of nanomaterials by splenic macrophages was found to be significant though less incisive than Kupffer cells. Nonetheless, spleen and liver Kupffer cells perform the same blood clearance activity, but they are size-sensitive. Indeed, as the NPs size exceed 200 nm, Kupffer cells uptake became less efficient and NPs capture by the spleen increase until reaching a maximum for particles larger than 400 nm [173]. Size selective splenic capture suggested that nanotheranostics could be formulated providing specific targeting for pathologies involving RES organs. One of the first report of passive spleen targeting by NPs drugs was proposed by Peracchia and co-workers who employed polymeric NPs which achieved specific ampicillin delivery to spleen, considerably reducing accumulation in the liver [174]. After that, a number of nanoformulations have been proposed for splenotropic delivery of drugs, including lipid NPs, polymeric NPs and chitosan NPs [175–177].

It is important to note that when the residence time of non-biodegradable nanomaterials, *e.g.* metal NPs, in the organism is prolonged, the likelihood of developing severe disorders is

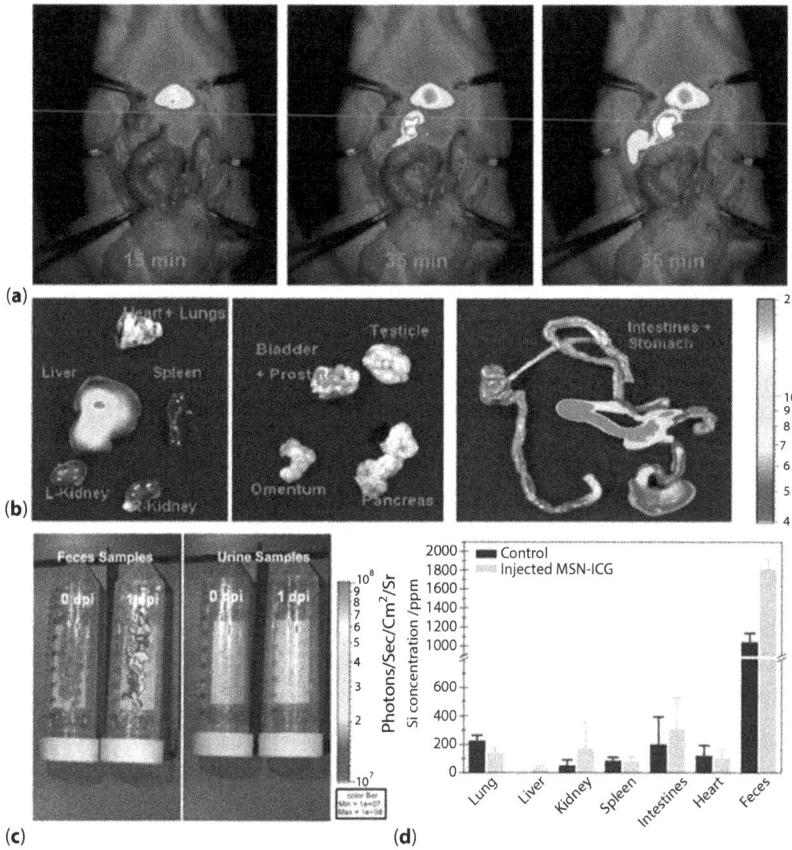

Figure 4.7 (a) Fluorescence imaging of silica NPs accumulating in mouse liver 15 minutes after systemic injection and subsequently migrating to the gastrointestinal tract. (b) *Ex vivo* fluorescence imaging of organs harvested from silica NPs treated mouse 3 hours after tail injection show NPs sequestration by the liver and migration in the intestine and stomach. (c) Fluorescence imaging of feces and urine collected from treated mouse respectively 0 days and 1 day after injection. (d) Presence of silicon in the feces is confirmed by mass spectroscopy analyses 3 days after NPs injection [180]. Reproduced from [180] with permission of Elsevier.

increased. For instance, albeit the toxicity of gold NPs is considered very low, gold is not significantly biodegraded by the organism, and hence its persistence in the organs could last for years [178]. This long-lasting accumulation of NPs has been the source of serious diseases including lysosomal disorders and autophagy, in which lysosomes were involved in intracellular organelles degradation, as they were recognized as foreign bodies due to the prolonged exposure to NPs. Alternatively, physiological autophagy was demonstrated to be blocked by the alkalinization of pH in the lysosomal compartment owing to the accumulation of gold NPs [179]. Hence it is important that administered nanomaterials are either degraded or excreted by the organism after having accomplished the therapeutic action. It has been demonstrated that liver has the capability of accumulating certain nanomaterials for a reasonable timeframe and get rid of them through excretion in the hepatobiliary route.

For instance, Souris and co-workers reported an interesting work in which they monitored the accumulation and excretion of dye-loaded silica nanomaterials in mice through fluorescence imaging and mass spectrometry analyses. The authors found an interesting dependence of the rate of excretion by the gastrointestinal tract from the surface charge of NPs. While a substantial amount of highly charged NPs was found in the feces, less charged ones remained sequestered within the liver, probably as a consequence of a differentiate opsonization occurred onto the surface of the nanomaterials (Figure 4.7) [180]. Similar results were found for micelle-encapsulated radiolabeled NPs of about 35 nm, which displayed preferential accumulation in the liver and efficient clearance through hepatobiliary routes in 72 hours [181].

Nevertheless, the fecal excretion pathway has shown some concerns regarding its effectiveness and quickness. In a very recent report, it was revealed that hepatobiliary clearance of noble metal NPs of similar hydrodynamic diameter, in the range 12–15 nm, is material dependent and somehow inefficient. Gold and silver NPs were administered repeatedly to mice for 25 days and feces were analyzed during this period and for the following 30 days. They have observed a detectable, yet not conspicuous, fecal excretion for silver NPs but not detectable gold content was found during that timeframe, confirming the stable accumulation of gold in RES [182].

Renal Filtration

When discussing about systemic administration of inorganic NPs, in particular noble metal NPs, we have pointed out some issues related to their excretion from the RES via hepatobiliary route, which is a relatively slow and inefficient process. NPs with a size ranging from 10 nm to hundreds of nm are readily captured by macrophages and transported to liver and spleen, according to their size. Here, if not biodegradable, NPs tend to reside for an unacceptable period of time which is the cause of severe diseases. However, NPs whose diameter is smaller than 10 nm may suffer a different fate due to other organs competing with RES for the blood clearance in this size regime: the kidneys.

Kidneys serve as an efficient filter to passively remove materials in the bloodstream from the urinary system, as long as their size does not exceed the threshold of their anatomic barriers. Blood and urine filtration in the kidneys take place in their functional units, named nephrons, more specifically in their filtering component called renal corpuscle. The corpuscle is composed by a tangle of capillaries made of endothelial cells, called glomerulus, and the Bowman's capsule. Understanding the anatomy of the glomerulus clarifies the mechanisms and size threshold for renal excretion of nanomaterials. The glomerular filtration barrier separates the blood capillaries from Bowman's space, and is composed by a layer of endothelial cells that have fenestrations of 70–90 nm, a basement membrane and a layer of podocytes (Figure 4.8a). Since the basement membrane has holes of 2–8 nm and the podocytes are separated by slits of 4–11 nm, the combination of these apertures pose a size threshold for renal clearance to 6–8 nm [183]. It is straightforward to note that this size threshold does not refer to the physical diameter of the nanomaterials, yet to their *in vivo* hydrodynamic diameter. Thus, nanomaterials that can be successfully excreted by kidneys have a physical size that typically does not exceed 3 nm, that is the regime known as "ultrasmall" (ultrasmall nanoparticles, USNPs). Alternatively, NPs bigger than 3 nm can be excreted from the renal pathway only if biodegradable, and if the building blocks are smaller than the threshold size.

An outstanding investigation regarding the exact size over which renal filtration is impaired has been published in 2007 by Choi and co-workers. The authors synthesized quantum dots with precise hydrodynamic diameter in the range 4.36–8.65 nm

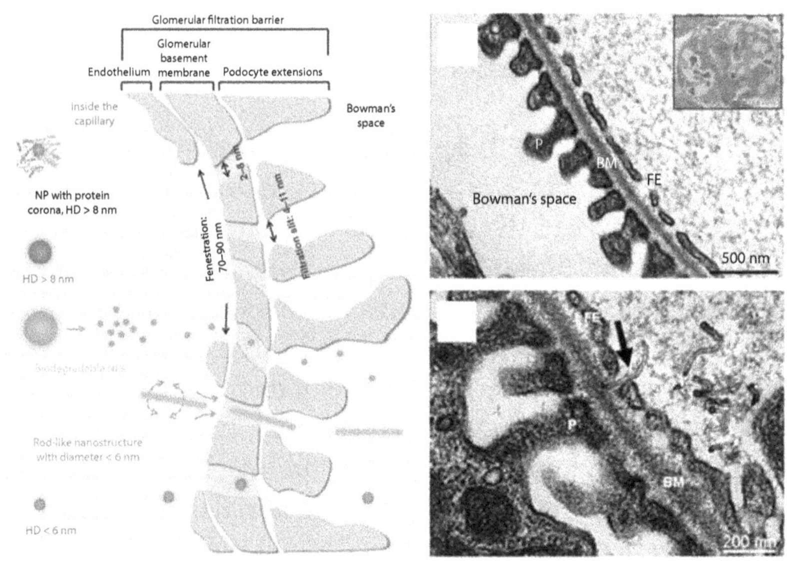

Figure 4.8 (a) Scheme of the glomerular filtration barrier separating the blood capillary from Bowman's space, showing the three components that dictate the size threshold for renal clearance: fenestrated endothelium, basement membrane and podocytes. (b) TEM images of glomerular filtration barrier in mice (top) showing that high aspect ratio carbon nanotubes can effectively cross the barrier and translocate to Bowman's space [183, 191]. (a) Reprinted from [183] with permission of John Wiley & Sons Inc. (b) Reprinted from [191] with permission of John Wiley & Sons Inc

by employing zwitterionic coatings for circumventing excessive protein adsorption. Quantum dots were administered through systemic injection to assess the excretion capability of kidneys, and it was finally defined a size threshold for the excretion of 5.5 nm [184]. Actually, previous findings on the pharmacokinetics of dendrimers on mouse models already suggested a similar threshold value albeit a precise size was not provided. Indeed, Kobayashi *et al.* observed that PAMAM dendrimers engineered to serve as MRI contrast agents were effectively cleared by kidneys as far as their diameter was below 6 nm [185]. Similarly, Zhou *et al.* performed biodistribution analyses in mice on glutathione-coated gold NPs of about 6 nm and 13 nm hydrodynamic diameter. They found that smaller NPs displayed an eightfold increase in renal excretion with respect to the bigger ones, and a substantial decrease in the accumulation in the RES [186]. Plenty of reports involving renal clearance of other nanomaterials including silica NPs, quantum dots, gold NPs, gadolinium and carbon based NPs, confirmed the threshold size for kidney filtration at 6 nm [187]. Interestingly, while optimal size for passive clearance via glomerular filtration seems to be established, it has been shown that NPs in the size range 6–8 nm can be also excreted by urines, yet their clearance is dictated by the surface charge. Indeed, glomerular basement membrane is negatively charged and hence facilitates the filtration of cationic NPs with respect to anionic ones of the same size, owing to electrostatic repulsion. Unexpectedly, Liang and co-workers published a work in which they investigated the pharmacokinetic profile of anionic quantum dots with a hydrodynamic diameter of 3.7 nm after intravenous injection. Being smaller than the filtration threshold, efficient renal clearance was expected, nevertheless these USNPs failed to be excreted, in contrast to their cationic counterpart of same size [188]. Similarly, another group found that negatively charged quantum dots whose hydrodynamic diameter was in the range 2.9–4.5 nm were also mainly accumulated in the kidney up to

80 days after systemic injection [189]. This effect should not be underestimated as it could produce unwanted accumulation in the kidneys instead of body excretion, ultimately leading to nephrotoxicity and disruption of kidney functions [190].

Another important step in understanding the rules of renal clearance was the finding that anisotropic nanomaterials with at least one dimension in the optimal size range for filtration were able to cross the glomerulus slits and be excreted. For instance, carbon nanotubes with average length from 300 to 1000 nm but whose diameter was around 1 nm were shown to achieve quick and effective renal clearance and excretion in the urines [192]. On this regard, Ruggiero and co-workers proposed a mathematical model that attempted an explanation to this behavior. They proposed that the blood flow in the glomerulus is enough to stir the nanotubes and align their major axis with the glomerular pores, thus allowing for effective translocation in the Bowman's space [193]. This effect was confirmed by TEM imaging of kidney sections of mice treated with carbon nanotubes, which clearly showed nanotubes that transversally crossed the basement membrane to reach Bowman's space (Figure 4.8b) [191]. Finally, another important finding regarding the size cutoff of the glomerular filtration barrier involves the renal clearance of sub-nanometric nanoparticles (*i.e.* clusters) and was very recently reported by Du *et al.* They investigated renal clearance kinetics of gold clusters made up by 10 to 25 gold atoms, whose size didn't exceed 1 nm. These particles displayed unique *in vivo* kinetics: in the sub-nanometric regime (from 10 to 18 gold atoms) the renal clearance efficiency was decreased from four- to nine-fold respect to clusters composed by 25 atoms [194]. Noteworthy, this peculiar behavior of the glomerular barrier which discerns few atoms difference in sub nanometric NPs may have deep implications in their passive targeting capability. It was speculated that the slow clearance profile of few-atoms NPs could in turn yield prolonged blood circulation time and impaired extravasation from normal vessels, hence enhancing their permeability and retention in cancer tissues.

Overall, nanomaterials interact with biological entities at multiple levels, also yielding harmful effects. In this chapter, we have discussed nanomaterials' behavior both at cellular level, reviewing the uptake pathways and cytotoxicity mechanisms, and at body level, from their administration by intravenous route, to their excretion through hepatobiliary routes. Understanding these mechanisms is an argument of paramount importance since the clinical success of nanomaterials is primarily determined by their biointeractions.

References

1. Kettiger, H., Schipanski, A., Wick, P. & Huwyler, J. Engineered nanomaterial uptake and tissue distribution: From cell to organism. *Int. J. Nanomedicine* 8, 3255–3269, 2013.
2. Mayor, S. and Pagano R.E.,Pathways of clathrin-independent endocytosis. Nature Reviews Molecular Cell Biology 8, 603-612 (2007)
2. Lim, J. P. & Gleeson, P. A. Macropinocytosis: an endocytic pathway for internalising large gulps. *Immunol. Cell Biol.* 89, 836–843, 2011.
3. Williams, K. E. N. N. E. T. H. & B, L. J. Non-specific adsorptive pinocytosis. 527–528, 1983.
4. REJMAN, J., OBERLE, V., ZUHORN, I. S. & HOEKSTRA, D. Size-dependent internalization of particles via the pathways of clathrin- and caveolae-mediated endocytosis. *Biochem. J.* 377, 159–169, 2004.
5. Parayath, N. N. & Amiji, M. M. Therapeutic targeting strategies using endogenous cells and proteins. *J. Control. Release* 258, 81–94, 2017.
6. Wang, J., Tian, S., Petros, R. A., Napier, M. E. & DeSimone, J. M. The Complex Role of Multivalency in Nanoparticles Targeting the Transferrin Receptor for Cancer Therapies. *J. Am. Chem. Soc.* 132, 11306–11313, 2010.

7. Ulbrich, K., Hekmatara, T., Herbert, E. & Kreuter, J. Transferrin- and transferrin-receptor-antibody-modified nanoparticles enable drug delivery across the blood–brain barrier (BBB). *Eur. J. Pharm. Biopharm.* 71, 251–256, 2009.
8. Santi, M. *et al.* Rational Design of a Transferrin-Binding Peptide Sequence Tailored to Targeted Nanoparticle Internalization. *Bioconjug. Chem.* 28, 471–480, 2017.
9. Schubert, W. *et al.* Caveolae-deficient Endothelial Cells Show Defects in the Uptake and Transport of Albumin *In Vivo*. *J. Biol. Chem.* 276, 48619–48622, 2001.
10. Chatterjee, M. *et al.* Caveolae-Mediated Endocytosis is Critical for Albumin Cellular Uptake and Response to Albumin-Bound Chemotherapy. *Cancer Res.* 77(21), pp. 5925–5937, 2017.
11. Kou, L., Sun, J., Zhai, Y. & He, Z. The endocytosis and intracellular fate of nanomedicines: Implication for rational design. *Asian J. Pharm. Sci.* 8, 1–8, 2013.
12. Maxfield, F. R. & McGraw, T. E. Endocytic recycling. *Nat. Rev. Mol. Cell Biol.* 5, 121–132, 2004.
13. Szymanowski, F. *et al.* Endocytosis and intracellular traffic of cholesterol-PDMAEMA liposome complexes in human epithelial-like cells. *Colloids Surfaces B Biointerfaces* 156, 38–43, 2017.
14. Pelkmans, L., Kartenbeck, J. & Helenius, A. Caveolar endocytosis of simian virus 40 reveals a new two-step vesicular-transport pathway to the ER. *Nat. Cell Biol.* 3, 473–483, 2001.
15. Hayer, A. *et al.* Caveolin-1 is ubiquitinated and targeted to intralumenal vesicles in endolysosomes for degradation. *J. Cell Biol.* 191, 615–629, 2010.
16. Voigt, J., Christensen, J. & Shastri, V. P. Differential uptake of nanoparticles by endothelial cells through polyelectrolytes with affinity for caveolae. *Proc. Natl. Acad. Sci.* 111, 2942–2947, 2014.
17. Sundaramoorthy, P. *et al.* Engineering of caveolae-specific self-micellizing anticancer lipid nanoparticles to enhance the chemotherapeutic efficacy of oxaliplatin in colorectal cancer cells. *Acta Biomater.* 42, 220–231, 2016.
18. Behr, J. The proton sponge: a trick to enter cells the viruses did not exploit. *Int. J. Chem.* 2, 34–36, 1997.

19. Lu, S., Morris, V. B. & Labhasetwar, V. Codelivery of DNA and siRNA via Arginine-Rich PEI-Based Polyplexes. *Mol. Pharm.* 12, 621–629, 2015.
20. Noh, S. M. *et al.* Pegylated poly-l-arginine derivatives of chitosan for effective delivery of siRNA. *J. Control. Release* 145, 159–164, 2010.
21. Liu, X. *et al.* Promoting siRNA delivery via enhanced cellular uptake using an arginine-decorated amphiphilic dendrimer. *Nanoscale* 7, 3867–3875, 2015.
22. Li, J. *et al.* Copolymer of poly(ethylene glycol) and poly(L-lysine) grafting polyethylenimine through a reducible disulfide linkage for siRNA delivery. *Nanoscale* 6, 1732–1740, 2014.
23. Zhao, Z.-X. *et al.* Self-assembly nanomicelles based on cationic mPEG-PLA-b-Polyarginine(R15) triblock copolymer for siRNA delivery. *Biomaterials* 33, 6793–6807, 2012.
24. Won, Y. Y., Sharma, R. & Konieczny, S. F. Missing pieces in understanding the intracellular trafficking of polycation/DNA complexes. *J. Control. Release* 139, 88–93, 2009.
25. Cheng, Y., Yumul, R. C. & Pun, S. H. Virus-Inspired Polymer for Efficient *In Vitro* and *In Vivo* Gene Delivery. *Angew. Chemie Int. Ed.* 55, 12013–12017, 2016.
26. Frankel, A. D. & Pabo, C. O. Cellular uptake of the tat protein from human immunodeficiency virus. *Cell* 55, 1189–1193, 1988.
27. Lo, S. L. & Wang, S. An endosomolytic Tat peptide produced by incorporation of histidine and cysteine residues as a nonviral vector for DNA transfection. *Biomaterials* 29, 2408–2414, 2008.
28. Ferrari, A. *et al.* Caveolae-mediated internalization of extracellular HIV-1 tat fusion proteins visualized in real time. *Mol. Ther.* 8, 284–94, 2003.
29. Wadia, J. S., Stan, R. V & Dowdy, S. F. Transducible TAT-HA fusogenic peptide enhances escape of TAT-fusion proteins after lipid raft macropinocytosis. *Nat. Med.* 10, 310–315, 2004.
30. Salomone, F. *et al.* A novel chimeric cell-penetrating peptide with membrane-disruptive properties for efficient endosomal escape. *J. Control. Release* 163, 293–303, 2012.

31. Albanese, A., Tang, P. S. & Chan, W. C. W. The Effect of Nanoparticle Size, Shape, and Surface Chemistry on Biological Systems. *Annu. Rev. Biomed. Eng.* 14, 1–16, 2012.
32. Chithrani, B. D., Ghazani, A. A. & Chan, W. C. W. Determining the size and shape dependence of gold nanoparticle uptake into mammalian cells. *Nano Lett.* 6, 662–668, 2006.
33. Chithrani, B. D. & Chan, W. C. Elucidating the mechanism of cellular uptake and removal of protein-coated gold nanoparticles of different sizes and shapes. TL - 7. *Nano Lett.* 7 **VN-re,** 1542–1550, 2007.
34. Zhu, J. *et al.* Size-dependent cellular uptake efficiency, mechanism, and cytotoxicity of silica nanoparticles toward HeLa cells. *Talanta* 107, 408–415, 2013.
35. Lu, F., Wu, S.-H., Hung, Y. & Mou, C.-Y. Size Effect on Cell Uptake in Well-Suspended, Uniform Mesoporous Silica Nanoparticles. *Small* 5, 1408–1413, 2009.
36. Varela, J. A., Bexiga, M. G., Åberg, C., Simpson, J. C. & Dawson, K. A. Quantifying size-dependent interactions between fluorescently labeled polystyrene nanoparticles and mammalian cells. *J. Nanobiotechnology* 10, 39, 2012.
37. Huang, J. *et al.* Effects of Nanoparticle Size on Cellular Uptake and Liver MRI with PVP-Coated Iron Oxide Nanoparticles. *ACS Nano* 4, 7151–7160, 2010.
38. Arnida, Janát-Amsbury, M. M., Ray, A., Peterson, C. M. & Ghandehari, H. Geometry and surface characteristics of gold nanoparticles influence their biodistribution and uptake by macrophages. *Eur. J. Pharm. Biopharm.* 77, 417–423, 2011.
39. Meng, H. *et al.* Aspect Ratio Determines the Quantity of Mesoporous Silica Nanoparticle Uptake by a Small GTPase-Dependent Macropinocytosis Mechanism. *ACS Nano* 5, 4434–4447, 2011.
40. Florez, L. *et al.* How Shape Influences Uptake: Interactions of Anisotropic Polymer Nanoparticles and Human Mesenchymal Stem Cells. *Small* 8, 2222–2230, 2012.
41. Vácha, R., Martinez-Veracoechea, F. J. & Frenkel, D. Receptor-Mediated Endocytosis of Nanoparticles of Various Shapes. *Nano Lett.* 11, 5391–5395, 2011.

42. Dasgupta, S., Auth, T. & Gompper, G. Shape and Orientation Matter for the Cellular Uptake of Nonspherical Particles. *Nano Lett.* 14, 687–693, 2014.
43. Fröhlich, E. The role of surface charge in cellular uptake and cytotoxicity of medical nanoparticles. *Int. J. Nanomedicine* 7: 5577–5591, 2012.
44. Miller, C. R., Bondurant, B., McLean, S. D., McGovern, K. A. & O'Brien, D. F. Liposome–Cell Interactions *in Vitro*: Effect of Liposome Surface Charge on the Binding and Endocytosis of Conventional and Sterically Stabilized Liposomes. *Biochemistry* 37, 12875–12883, 1998.
45. Marquis, B. J., Liu, Z., Braun, K. L. & Haynes, C. L. Investigation of noble metal nanoparticleζ-potential effects on single-cell exocytosis function *in vitro* with carbon-fiber microelectrode amperometry. *Analyst* 136, 3478–3486, 2011.
46. Villanueva, A. *et al.* The influence of surface functionalization on the enhanced internalization of magnetic nanoparticles in cancer cells. *Nanotechnology* 20, 115103, 2009.
47. Chung, T.-H. *et al.* The effect of surface charge on the uptake and biological function of mesoporous silica nanoparticles in 3T3-L1 cells and human mesenchymal stem cells. *Biomaterials* 28, 2959–2966, 2007.
48. Lunov, O. *et al.* Differential Uptake of Functionalized Polystyrene Nanoparticles by Human Macrophages and a Monocytic Cell Line. *ACS Nano* 5, 1657–1669, 2011.
49. Yue, Z.-G. *et al.* Surface Charge Affects Cellular Uptake and Intracellular Trafficking of Chitosan-Based Nanoparticles. *Biomacromolecules* 12, 2440–2446, 2011.
50. Leroueil, P. R. *et al.* Wide Varieties of Cationic Nanoparticles Induce Defects in Supported Lipid Bilayers. *Nano Lett.* 8, 420–424, 2008.
51. Lin, J. & Alexander-Katz, A. Cell Membranes Open 'Doors' for Cationic Nanoparticles/Biomolecules: Insights into Uptake Kinetics. *ACS Nano* 7, 10799–10808, 2013.
52. Bhatia, S. K. & Yetter, A. B. Correlation of visual *in vitro* cytotoxicity ratings of biomaterials with quantitative *in vitro* cell viability measurements. *Cell Biol. Toxicol.* 24, 315–319, 2008.

53. Fiorito, S., Serafino, A., Andreola, F. & Bernier, P. Effects of fullerenes and single-wall carbon nanotubes on murine and human macrophages. *Carbon N. Y.* 44, 1100–1105, 2006.
54. Marquis, B. J., Love, S. A., Braun, K. L. & Haynes, C. L. Analytical methods to assess nanoparticle toxicity. *Analyst* 134, 425, 2009.
55. Lewinski, N., Colvin, V. & Drezek, R. Cytotoxicity of Nanoparticles. *Small* 4, 26–49, 2008.
56. Thompson T.A., *Neurodegeneration Methods and Protocols. Methods in Molecular Medicine™*, vol 22. pp 145–156, Humana Press, NJ. 1999.
57. Thomas, M. & Klibanov, A. M. Conjugation to gold nanoparticles enhances polyethylenimine's transfer of plasmid DNA into mammalian cells. *Proc. Natl. Acad. Sci.* 100, 9138–9143, 2003.
58. Takahashi, H. *et al.* Modification of Gold Nanorods Using Phosphatidylcholine to Reduce Cytotoxicity. *Langmuir* 22, 2–5, 2006.
59. Connor, E. E., Mwamuka, J., Gole, A., Murphy, C. J. & Wyatt, M. D. Gold Nanoparticles Are Taken Up by Human Cells but Do Not Cause Acute Cytotoxicity. *Small* 1, 325–327, 2005.
60. Petri-Fink, A., Chastellain, M., Juillerat-Jeanneret, L., Ferrari, A. & Hofmann, H. Development of functionalized superparamagnetic iron oxide nanoparticles for interaction with human cancer cells. *Biomaterials* 26, 2685–2694, 2005.
61. CHENG, F. et. al. Characterization of aqueous dispersions of Fe3O4 nanoparticles and their biomedical applications. *Biomaterials* 26, 729–738, 2005.
62. Derfus, A. M., Chan, W. C. W. & Bhatia, S. N. Probing the Cytotoxicity of Semiconductor Quantum Dots. *Nano Lett.* 4, 11–18, 2004.
63. Duan, H. & Nie, S. Cell-Penetrating Quantum Dots Based on Multivalent and Endosome-Disrupting Surface Coatings. *J. Am. Chem. Soc.* 129, 3333–3338, 2007.
64. Jia, G. *et al.* Cytotoxicity of carbon nanomaterials: single-wall nanotube, multi-wall nanotube, and fullerene. *Environ. Sci. Technol.* 39, 1378–83, 2005.
65. Magrez, A. *et al.* Cellular Toxicity of Carbon-Based Nanomaterials. *Nano Lett.* 6, 1121–1125, 2006.

66. Martina, M.-S. *et al.* Generation of Superparamagnetic Liposomes Revealed as Highly Efficient MRI Contrast Agents for *in Vivo* Imaging. *J. Am. Chem. Soc.* 127, 10676–10685, 2005.
67. Tominaga, H. *et al.* A water-soluble tetrazolium salt useful for colorimetric cell viability assay. *Anal. Commun.* 36, 47–50, 1999.
68. Kong, B., Seog, J. H., Graham, L. M. & Lee, S. B. Experimental considerations on the cytotoxicity of nanoparticles. *Nanomedicine* 6, 929–941, 2011.
69. Angius, F. & Floris, A. Liposomes and MTT cell viability assay: An incompatible affair. *Toxicol. Vitr.* 29, 314–319, 2015.
70. Altunbek, M. & Culha, M. Influence of Plasmonic Nanoparticles on the Performance of Colorimetric Cell Viability Assays. *Plasmonics* 12, 1749–1760, 2017.
71. Vinković Vrček, I. *et al.* Does surface coating of metallic nanoparticles modulate their interference with *in vitro* assays? *RSC Adv.* 5, 70787–70807, 2015.
72. Lupu, A. R. & Popescu, T. The noncellular reduction of MTT tetrazolium salt by TiO2 nanoparticles and its implications for cytotoxicity assays. *Toxicol. Vitr.* 27, 1445–1450, 2013.
73. Fisichella, M. *et al.* Mesoporous silica nanoparticles enhance MTT formazan exocytosis in HeLa cells and astrocytes. *Toxicol. Vitr.* 23, 697–703, 2009.
74. Panda, K. K. *et al. In vitro* biosynthesis and genotoxicity bioassay of silver nanoparticles using plants. *Toxicol. Vitr.* 25, 1097–1105, 2011.
75. Asare, N. *et al.* Cytotoxic and genotoxic effects of silver nanoparticles in testicular cells. *Toxicology* 291, 65–72, 2012.
76. Hackenberg, S. *et al.* Silver nanoparticles: Evaluation of DNA damage, toxicity and functional impairment in human mesenchymal stem cells. *Toxicol. Lett.* 201, 27–33, 2011.
77. Flower, N. A. L. *et al.* Characterization of synthesized silver nanoparticles and assessment of its genotoxicity potentials using the alkaline comet assay. *Mutat. Res. Toxicol. Environ. Mutagen.* 742, 61–65, 2012.
78. AshaRani, P. V., Low Kah Mun, G., Hande, M. P. & Valiyaveettil, S. Cytotoxicity and Genotoxicity of Silver Nanoparticles in Human Cells. *ACS Nano* 3, 279–290, 2009.

79. Kim, H. R., Kim, M. J., Lee, S. Y., Oh, S. M. & Chung, K. H. Genotoxic effects of silver nanoparticles stimulated by oxidative stress in human normal bronchial epithelial (BEAS-2B) cells. *Mutat. Res. Toxicol. Environ. Mutagen.* 726, 129–135, 2011.
80. Liman, R. Genotoxic effects of Bismuth (III) oxide nanoparticles by Allium and Comet assay. *Chemosphere* 93, 269–273, 2013.
81. Sharma, V., Anderson, D. & Dhawan, A. Zinc Oxide Nanoparticles Induce Oxidative Stress and Genotoxicity in Human Liver Cells (HepG2). *J. Biomed. Nanotechnol.* 7, 98–99, 2011.
82. Bhattacharya, K. *et al.* Titanium dioxide nanoparticles induce oxidative stress and DNA-adduct formation but not DNA-breakage in human lung cells. *Part. Fibre Toxicol.* 6, 17, 2009.
83. Shukla, R. K. *et al.* TiO 2 nanoparticles induce oxidative DNA damage and apoptosis in human liver cells. *Nanotoxicology* 7, 48–60, 2013.
84. Barnes, C. A. *et al.* Reproducible Comet Assay of Amorphous Silica Nanoparticles Detects No Genotoxicity. *Nano Lett.* 8, 3069–3074, 2008.
85. Magdolenova, Z. *et al.* Mechanisms of genotoxicity. A review of *in vitro* and *in vivo* studies with engineered nanoparticles. *Nanotoxicology* 8, 233–278, 2014.
86. Yildirimer, L., Thanh, N. T. K., Loizidou, M. & Seifalian, A. M. Toxicology and clinical potential of nanoparticles. *Nano Today* 6, 585–607, 2011.
87. Aggarwal, P., Hall, J. B., McLeland, C. B., Dobrovolskaia, M. A. & McNeil, S. E. Nanoparticle interaction with plasma proteins as it relates to particle biodistribution, biocompatibility and therapeutic efficacy. *Adv. Drug Deliv. Rev.* 61, 428–437, 2009.
88. Piella, J., Bastús, N. G. & Puntes, V. Size-Dependent Protein–Nanoparticle Interactions in Citrate-Stabilized Gold Nanoparticles: The Emergence of the Protein Corona. *Bioconjug. Chem.* 28, 88–97, 2017.
89. Bertrand, N. *et al.* Mechanistic understanding of *in vivo* protein corona formation on polymeric nanoparticles and impact on pharmacokinetics. *Nat. Commun.* 8, 777, 2017.
90. Lundqvist, M. *et al.* Nanoparticle size and surface properties determine the protein corona with possible implications for biological impacts. *Proc. Natl. Acad. Sci.* 105, 14265–14270, 2008.

91. Tenzer, S. *et al.* Nanoparticle size is a critical physicochemical determinant of the human blood plasma corona: A comprehensive quantitative proteomic analysis. *ACS Nano* 5, 7155–7167, 2011.
92. Dobrovolskaia, M. A., Aggarwal, P., Hall, J. B. & McNeil, S. E. Preclinical Studies To Understand Nanoparticle Interaction with the Immune System and Its Potential Effects on Nanoparticle Biodistribution. *Mol. Pharm.* 5, 487–495, 2008.
93. Mahmoudi, M. *et al.* Protein–Nanoparticle Interactions: Opportunities and Challenges. *Chem. Rev.* 111, 5610–5637, 2011.
94. Rio-Echevarria, I. M. *et al.* Highly PEGylated silica nanoparticles: 'ready to use' stealth functional nanocarriers. *J. Mater. Chem.* 20, 2780, 2010.
95. Klibanov, A. L., Maruyama, K., Torchilin, V. P. & Huang, L. Amphipathic polyethyleneglycols effectively prolong the circulation time of liposomes. *FEBS Lett.* 268, 235–237, 1990.
96. Gref, R. *et al.* Biodegradable long-circulating polymeric nanospheres. *Science (80-.).* 263, 1600–1603, 1994.
97. Niidome, T. *et al.* PEG-modified gold nanorods with a stealth character for *in vivo* applications. *J. Control. Release* 114, 343–347, 2006.
98. Yang, S. *et al.* Covalently PEGylated Carbon Nanotubes with Stealth Character *In Vivo*. *Small* 4, 940–944, 2008.
99. Stolnik, S. *et al.* Surface Modification of Poly(lactide-co-glycolide) Nanospheres by Biodegradable Poly(lactide)-Poly(ethylene glycol) Copolymers. *Pharm. Res.* 11, 1800–1808, 1994.
100. Barenholz, Y. (Chezy). Doxil® – The first FDA-approved nano-drug: Lessons learned. *J. Control. Release* 160, 117–134, 2012.
101. Dams, E. T. *et al.* Accelerated blood clearance and altered biodistribution of repeated injections of sterically stabilized liposomes. *J. Pharmacol. Exp. Ther.* 292, 1071–1079, 2000.
102. Mima, Y., Hashimoto, Y., Shimizu, T., Kiwada, H. & Ishida, T. Anti-PEG IgM Is a Major Contributor to the Accelerated Blood Clearance of Polyethylene Glycol-Conjugated Protein. *Mol. Pharm.* 12, 2429–2435, 2015.
103. MISHRA, S. PEGylation significantly affects cellular uptake and intracellular trafficking of non-viral gene delivery particles. *Eur. J. Cell Biol.* 83, 97–111, 2004.

104. Remaut, K., Lucas, B., Braeckmans, K., Demeester, J. & De Smedt, S. C. Pegylation of liposomes favours the endosomal degradation of the delivered phosphodiester oligonucleotides. *J. Control. Release* 117, 256–266, 2007.
105. Amoozgar, Z. & Yeo, Y. Recent advances in stealth coating of nanoparticle drug delivery systems. *Wiley Interdiscip. Rev. Nanomedicine Nanobiotechnology* 4, 219–233, 2012.
106. Sawant, R. M. *et al.* 'SMART' Drug Delivery Systems: Double-Targeted pH-Responsive Pharmaceutical Nanocarriers. *Bioconjug. Chem.* 17, 943–949, 2006.
107. Ranalli, A. *et al.* Peptide-Based Stealth Nanoparticles for Targeted and pH-Triggered Delivery. *Bioconjug. Chem.* 28, 627–635, 2017.
108. Parodi, A. *et al.* Synthetic nanoparticles functionalized with biomimetic leukocyte membranes possess cell-like functions. *Nat. Nanotechnol.* 8, 61–68, 2012.
109. El-Andaloussi, S. *et al.* Exosome-mediated delivery of siRNA *in vitro* and *in vivo*. *Nat. Protoc.* 7, 2112–2126, 2012.
110. Rother, R. P., Bell, L., Hillmen, P. & Gladwin, M. T. The Clinical Sequelae of Intravascular Hemolysis and Extracellular Plasma Hemoglobin. *JAMA* 293, 1653, 2005.
111. Chun, A. L. Silica nanoparticles: Keep the red stuff in. *Nat. Nanotechnol.*, 2008.
112. Chen, H.-T., Neerman, M. F., Parrish, A. R. & Simanek, E. E. Cytotoxicity, Hemolysis, and Acute *in Vivo* Toxicity of Dendrimers Based on Melamine, Candidate Vehicles for Drug Delivery. *J. Am. Chem. Soc.* 126, 10044–10048, 2004.
113. Ghosh, M., Chakraborty, A. & Mukherjee, A. Cytotoxic, genotoxic and the hemolytic effect of titanium dioxide (TiO 2) nanoparticles on human erythrocyte and lymphocyte cells *in vitro*. *J. Appl. Toxicol.* 33, 1097–1110, 2013.
114. Choi, J., Reipa, V., Hitchins, V. M., Goering, P. L. & Malinauskas, R. A. Physicochemical Characterization and *In Vitro* Hemolysis Evaluation of Silver Nanoparticles. *Toxicol. Sci.* 123, 133–143, 2011.
115. Trpkovic, A. *et al.* Oxidative stress-mediated hemolytic activity of solvent exchange-prepared fullerene (C 60) nanoparticles. *Nanotechnology* 21, 375102, 2010.

116. Fornaguera, C. *et al.* Interactions of PLGA nanoparticles with blood components: protein adsorption, coagulation, activation of the complement system and hemolysis studies. *Nanoscale* 7, 6045–6058, 2015.
117. Yildirim, A., Ozgur, E. & Bayindir, M. Impact of mesoporous silica nanoparticle surface functionality on hemolytic activity, thrombogenicity and non-specific protein adsorption. *J. Mater. Chem. B* 1, 1909, 2013.
118. Durgadas, C. V., Kaladhar, K., Divya, P., Sreenivasan, K. & Sharma, C. P. Preliminary Studies on Blood Compatibility and Langmuir Monolayer Stability of Gold Nanoparticles Stabilized Through Amino-PEG Functionality. *Trends Biomater. Artif. Organs* 23, 86–92, 2009.
119. Saha, K., Moyano, D. F. & Rotello, V. M. Protein coronas suppress the hemolytic activity of hydrophilic and hydrophobic nanoparticles. *Mater. Horiz.* 1, 102–105, 2014.
120. Toy, R., Hayden, E., Shoup, C., Baskaran, H. & Karathanasis, E. The effects of particle size, density and shape on margination of nanoparticles in microcirculation. *Nanotechnology* 22, 115101, 2011.
121. Lee, S.-Y., Ferrari, M. & Decuzzi, P. Shaping nano-/microparticles for enhanced vascular interaction in laminar flows. *Nanotechnology* 20, 495101, 2009.
122. Nadeem, S. & Ijaz, S. Influence of Metallic Nanoparticles on Blood Flow Through Arteries Having Both Stenosis and Aneurysm. *IEEE Trans. Nanobioscience* 14, 668–679, 2015.
123. Gentile, F. *et al.* The effect of shape on the margination dynamics of non-neutrally buoyant particles in two-dimensional shear flows. *J. Biomech.* 41, 2312–2318, 2008.
124. Doshi, N. *et al.* Flow and adhesion of drug carriers in blood vessels depend on their shape: A study using model synthetic microvascular networks. *J. Control. Release* 146, 196–200, 2010.
125. Toy, R., Peiris, P. M., Ghaghada, K. B. & Karathanasis, E. Shaping cancer nanomedicine: the effect of particle shape on the *in vivo* journey of nanoparticles. *Nanomedicine* 9, 121–134, 2014.
126. Tang, S. *et al.* Tailoring Renal Clearance and Tumor Targeting of Ultrasmall Metal Nanoparticles with Particle Density. *Angew. Chemie Int. Ed.* 55, 16039–16043, 2016.

127. Tan, J., Shah, S., Thomas, A., Ou-Yang, H. D. & Liu, Y. The influence of size, shape and vessel geometry on nanoparticle distribution. *Microfluid. Nanofluidics* 14, 77–87, 2013.
128. Skinner, S. A., Tutton, P. J. M. & O'Brien, P. E. Microvascular Architecture of Experimental Colon Tumors in the Rat. *Cancer Res.* 50, 2411–2417, 1990.
129. Sarin, H. Physiologic upper limits of pore size of different blood capillary types and another perspective on the dual pore theory of microvascular permeability. *J. Angiogenes. Res.* 2, 14, 2010.
130. Rippe, B. & Haraldsson, B. Transport of macromolecules across microvascular walls: the two-pore theory. *Physiol. Rev.* 74, 163–219, 1994.
131. Iyer, A. K., Khaled, G., Fang, J. & Maeda, H. Exploiting the enhanced permeability and retention effect for tumor targeting. *Drug Discov. Today* 11, 812–818, 2006.
132. Konno, T. *et al.* Selective targeting of anti-cancer drug and simultaneous image enhancement in solid tumors by arterially administered lipid contrast medium. *Cancer* 54, 2367–2374, 1984.
133. Matsumura, Y. & Maeda, H. A new concept for macromolecular therapeutics in cancer chemotherapy: mechanism of tumoritropic accumulation of proteins and the antitumor agent smancs. *Cancer Res.* 46, 6387–92, 1986.
134. Kopecek, J., Kopeckova, P., Minko, T. & Lu, Z.-R. HPMA copolymer–anticancer drug conjugates: design, activity, and mechanism of action. *Eur. J. Pharm. Biopharm.* 50, 61–81, 2000.
135. Uchino, H. *et al.* Cisplatin-incorporating polymeric micelles (NC-6004) can reduce nephrotoxicity and neurotoxicity of cisplatin in rats. *Br. J. Cancer* 93, 678–687, 2005.
136. Leu, A. J., Berk, D. A., Lymboussaki, A., Alitalo, K. & Jain, R. K. Absence of functional lymphatics within a murine sarcoma: a molecular and functional evaluation. *Cancer Res.* 60, 4324–7, 2000.
137. Omidi, Y. & Barar, J. Targeting tumor microenvironment: crossing tumor interstitial fluid by multifunctional nanomedicines. *Bioimpacts* 4, 55–67, 2014.
138. Lammers, T., Kiessling, F., Hennink, W. E. & Storm, G. Drug targeting to tumors: Principles, pitfalls and (pre-) clinical progress. *J. Control. Release* 161, 175–187, 2012.

139. Danhier, F. To exploit the tumor microenvironment: Since the EPR effect fails in the clinic, what is the future of nanomedicine? *J. Control. Release* 244, 108–121, 2016.
140. Carmeliet, P. VEGF as a Key Mediator of Angiogenesis in Cancer. *Oncology* 69, 4–10, 2005.
141. Nichols, J. W. & Bae, Y. H. EPR: Evidence and fallacy. *J. Control. Release* 190, 451–464, 2014.
142. Taurin, S., Nehoff, H. & Greish, K. Anticancer nanomedicine and tumor vascular permeability; Where is the missing link? *J. Control. Release* 164, 265–275, 2012.
144. Natfji, A. A., Ravishankar, D., Osborn, H. M. I. & Greco, F. Parameters Affecting the Enhanced Permeability and Retention Effect: The Need for Patient Selection. *J. Pharm. Sci.* 106, 3179–3187, 2017.
145. Nakamura, Y., Mochida, A., Choyke, P. L. & Kobayashi, H. Nanodrug Delivery: Is the Enhanced Permeability and Retention Effect Sufficient for Curing Cancer? *Bioconjug. Chem.* 27, 2225–2238, 2016.
146. Monsky, W. L. *et al.* Augmentation of transvascular transport of macromolecules and nanoparticles in tumors using vascular endothelial growth factor. *Cancer Res.* 59, 4129–35, 1999.
147. Tong, R. T. *et al.* Vascular Normalization by Vascular Endothelial Growth Factor Receptor 2 Blockade Induces a Pressure Gradient Across the Vasculature and Improves Drug Penetration in Tumors. *Cancer Res.* 64, 3731–3736, 2004.
148. Dickson, P. V. *et al.* Bevacizumab-Induced Transient Remodeling of the Vasculature in Neuroblastoma Xenografts Results in Improved Delivery and Efficacy of Systemically Administered Chemotherapy. *Clin. Cancer Res.* 13, 3942–3950, 2007.
149. Farrera, C. & Fadeel, B. It takes two to tango: Understanding the interactions between engineered nanomaterials and the immune system. *Eur. J. Pharm. Biopharm.* 95, 3–12, 2015.
150. Dobrovolskaia, M. A. & McNeil, S. E. Immunological properties of engineered nanomaterials. *Nat. Nanotechnol.* 2, 469–478, 2007.
151. Roberts, J. C., Bhalgat, M. K. & Zera, R. T. Preliminary biological evaluation of polyamidoamine (PAMAM) Starburst dendrimers. *J. Biomed. Mater. Res.* 30, 53–65, 1996.

152. Tomii, A. & Masugi, F. Production of anti-platelet-activating factor antibodies by the use of colloidal gold as carrier. *Jpn. J. Med. Sci. Biol.* 44, 75–80, 1991.
153. Oliveira, E. *et al.* Transcriptomic response of zebrafish embryos to polyaminoamine (PAMAM) dendrimers. *Nanotoxicology* 8, 92–99, 2014.
154. Palomäki, J., Karisola, P., Pylkkänen, L., Savolainen, K. & Alenius, H. Engineered nanomaterials cause cytotoxicity and activation on mouse antigen presenting cells. *Toxicology* 267, 125–131, 2010.
155. Chen, B. X., Wilson, S. R., Das, M., Coughlin, D. J. & Erlanger, B. F. Antigenicity of fullerenes: antibodies specific for fullerenes and their characteristics. *Proc. Natl. Acad. Sci. U. S. A.* 95, 10809–13, 1998.
156. Ilinskaya, A. N. & Dobrovolskaia, M. A. Understanding the immunogenicity and antigenicity of nanomaterials: Past, present and future. *Toxicol. Appl. Pharmacol.* 299, 70–7, 2016.
157. Watanabe, H., Nakanishi, T., Umetsu, M. & Kumagai, I. Human Anti-gold Antibodies. *J. Biol. Chem.* 283, 36031–36038, 2008.
158. Moyano, D. F. *et al.* Nanoparticle Hydrophobicity Dictates Immune Response. *J. Am. Chem. Soc.* 134, 3965–3967, 2012.
159. Keenan, B. P., Jaffee, E. M. & Armstrong, T. D. Tumor Immunology: Multidisciplinary Science Driving Basic and Clinical Advances. *Cancer Immunol. Res.* 1, 16–23, 2013.
160. Chakraborty, B. *et al.* Immunomodulatory properties of silver nanoparticles contribute to anticancer strategy for murine fibrosarcoma. *Cell. Mol. Immunol.* 13, 191–205, 2016.
161. Saptarshi, S. R., Duschl, A. & Lopata, A. L. Interaction of nanoparticles with proteins: relation to bio-reactivity of the nanoparticle. *J. Nanobiotechnology* 11, 26, 2013.
162. Deng, Z. J., Liang, M., Monteiro, M., Toth, I. & Minchin, R. F. Nanoparticle-induced unfolding of fibrinogen promotes Mac-1 receptor activation and inflammation. *Nat. Nanotechnol.* 6, 39–44, 2011.
163. Neagu, M. *et al.* Protein bio-corona: critical issue in immune nanotoxicology. *Arch. Toxicol.* 91, 1031–1048, 2017.
164. Wilhelm, S. *et al.* Analysis of nanoparticle delivery to tumours. *Nat. Rev. Mater.* 1, 16014, 2016.

165. De Jong, W. H. *et al.* Particle size-dependent organ distribution of gold nanoparticles after intravenous administration. *Biomaterials* 29, 1912–1919, 2008.
166. Terentyuk, G. S. *et al.* Circulation and distribution of gold nanoparticles and induced alterations of tissue morphology at intravenous particle delivery. *J. Biophotonics* 2, 292–302, 2009.
167. Zeng, J. *et al.* *In situ*111In-doping for achieving biocompatible and non-leachable 111In-labeled Fe3O4 nanoparticles. *Chem. Commun.* 50, 2170, 2014.
168. Huang, X. *et al.* The shape effect of mesoporous silica nanoparticles on biodistribution, clearance, and biocompatibility *in vivo*. *ACS Nano* 5, 5390–5399, 2011.
169. Zhao, Y. *et al.* A comparison between sphere and rod nanoparticles regarding their *in vivo* biological behavior and pharmacokinetics. *Sci. Rep.* 7, 4131, 2017.
170. Jenne, C. N. & Kubes, P. Immune surveillance by the liver. *Nat. Immunol.* 14, 996–1006, 2013.
171. Crean, P. A. *et al.* The fractional distribution of the cardiac output in man using microspheres labelled with technetium 99m. *Br. J. Radiol.* 59, 209–215, 1986.
172. Cataldi, M., Vigliotti, C., Mosca, T., Cammarota, M. & Capone, D. Emerging Role of the Spleen in the Pharmacokinetics of Monoclonal Antibodies, Nanoparticles and Exosomes. *Int. J. Mol. Sci.* 18, 1249, 2017.
173. Peracchia, M.. *et al.* Stealth® PEGylated polycyanoacrylate nanoparticles for intravenous administration and splenic targeting. *J. Control. Release* 60, 121–128, 1999.
174. Veerareddy, P. R., Vobalaboina, V. & Ali, N. Antileishmanial activity, pharmacokinetics and tissue distribution studies of mannose-grafted amphotericin B lipid nanospheres. *J. Drug Target.* 17, 140–147, 2009.
175. Ahmad, Z., Pandey, R., Sharma, S. & Khuller, G. K. Novel chemotherapy for tuberculosis: chemotherapeutic potential of econazole- and moxifloxacin-loaded PLG nanoparticles. *Int. J. Antimicrob. Agents* 31, 142–146, 2008.
176. Chaubey, P. & Mishra, B. Mannose-conjugated chitosan nanoparticles loaded with rifampicin for the treatment of visceral leishmaniasis. *Carbohydr. Polym.* 101, 1101–1108, 2014.

177. Khlebtsov, N. & Dykman, L. Biodistribution and toxicity of engineered gold nanoparticles: a review of *in vitro* and *in vivo* studies. *Chem. Soc. Rev.* 40, 1647–1671, 2011.
178. Ma, X. *et al.* Gold Nanoparticles Induce Autophagosome Accumulation through Size-Dependent Nanoparticle Uptake and Lysosome Impairment. *ACS Nano* 5, 8629–8639, 2011.
179. Souris, J. S. *et al.* Surface charge-mediated rapid hepatobiliary excretion of mesoporous silica nanoparticles. *Biomaterials* 31, 5564–5574, 2010.
180. Seo, H. J. *et al.* Rapid Hepatobiliary Excretion of Micelle-Encapsulated/Radiolabeled Upconverting Nanoparticles as an Integrated Form. *Sci. Rep.* 5, 15685, 2015.
181. Yang, L. *et al.* Comparisons of the biodistribution and toxicological examinations after repeated intravenous administration of silver and gold nanoparticles in mice. *Sci. Rep.* 7, 3303, 2017.
182. Xu, J., Peng, C., Yu, M. & Zheng, J. Renal clearable noble metal nanoparticles: photoluminescence, elimination, and biomedical applications. *Wiley Interdiscip. Rev. Nanomedicine Nanobiotechnology* 9, e1453, 2017.
183. Choi, H. S. *et al.* Renal clearance of quantum dots. *Nat. Biotechnol.* 25, 1165–1170, 2007.
184. KOBAYASHI, H. & BRECHBIEL, M. Nano-sized MRI contrast agents with dendrimer cores. *Adv. Drug Deliv. Rev.* 57, 2271–2286, 2005.
185. Zhou, C., Long, M., Qin, Y., Sun, X. & Zheng, J. Luminescent gold nanoparticles with efficient renal clearance. *Angew. Chemie - Int. Ed.* 50, 3168–3172, 2011.
186. Zarschler, K. *et al.* Ultrasmall inorganic nanoparticles: state-of-the-art and perspectives for biomedical applications. *Nanomedicine Nanotechnology, Biol. Med.* 12, 1663–1701, 2016.
187. Liang, X. *et al.* Short- and Long-Term Tracking of Anionic Ultrasmall Nanoparticles in Kidney. *ACS Nano* 10, 387–395, 2016.
188. Su, Y. *et al.* *In vivo* distribution, pharmacokinetics, and toxicity of aqueous synthesized cadmium-containing quantum dots. *Biomaterials* 32, 5855–5862, 2011.
189. Yamagishi, Y. *et al.* Acute and chronic nephrotoxicity of platinum nanoparticles in mice. *Nanoscale Res. Lett.* 8, 395, 2013.

190. Lacerda, L. *et al.* Carbon-Nanotube Shape and Individualization Critical for Renal Excretion. *Small* 4, 1130–1132, 2008.
191. Singh, R. *et al.* Tissue biodistribution and blood clearance rates of intravenously administered carbon nanotube radiotracers. *Proc. Natl. Acad. Sci.* 103, 3357–3362, 2006.
192. Ruggiero, A. *et al.* Paradoxical glomerular filtration of carbon nanotubes. *Proc. Natl. Acad. Sci.* 107, 12369–12374, 2010.
193. Du, B. *et al.* Glomerular barrier behaves as an atomically precise bandpass filter in a sub-nanometre regime. *Nat. Nanotechnol.* 12, 1096–1102, 2017.
194. Mayor, S. and Pagano R.E.,Pathways of clathrin-independent endocytosis. *Nature Reviews Molecular Cell Biology* 8, 603–612 2007.

5

Nanomaterials in the Market or in the Way of

In the last decades nanomaterials development have deeply revolutionized the way medicine is intended to be, shifting the therapeutic paradigm to personalized medicine, *i.e.* precise therapeutic plans tailored on each patient. In the previous chapters, we have discussed the unique benefits brought by nanomaterials to medicine as both therapeutic and diagnostic tools. On one hand, some researchers have focused their work on increasing the complexity of nanomaterials, producing single theranostics able to afford simultaneously multiple diagnostics modalities and controlled therapeutics delivery. Nevertheless, the step from the laboratory bench to the market is not obvious, and it gets harder by increasing the complexity of nanomaterials. Indeed, against the huge amount of published reports regarding nanotheranostics, only about 200 products have been clinically approved or are under clinical investigation [1]. Ideally, approved nanomedicines have been engineered in order to provide higher clinical benefit with respect to the standard-of-care and they had to overcome a series of rigid safety regulations that agencies such as U.S. food and drug administration (FDA) or European medicine agency (EMA) pose to safeguard patients' health. For instance, most of the clinically available nano-chemotherapeutics yield reduced toxicity and adverse effects with respect to classical drugs rather than increasing their therapeutic efficiency, yet this benefit has been sufficient to ensure their clinical translation. In this chapter, we deal with nanomaterials that have passed these regulations entering the commercial market for human use, or that are currently under investigation and have the potential to accomplish the translation from the bench to the bedside.

5.1 Approval Pipeline (FDA and EMA)

Regulation of the approval of new drugs and/or medical devices in the market is not a trivial task. The new product has to be assessed regarding safety and effectiveness as rapidly as possible. The translation pipeline of a new drug begins with a complete report of manufacturing specifications and preclinical data arguing the safety and efficacy of the new drug in animal models. Then the competent organ, *e.g.* FDA, enable an investigational new drug application (IND), that is the phase preceding clinical trials, in which the agency has 30 days to assess if the new product is reasonably safe for human tests [2]. After IND approbation, the new drug has to face three phases of clinical trials before being eventually placed on the market (Figure 5.1). Phase I involves about 20-100 healthy volunteers or patients bearing life-threatening illness, which are constantly monitored to evaluate safety and pharmacology of the product, which is however administered at low dosage. Usually, the very next step in phase I is estimating the lowest drug amount

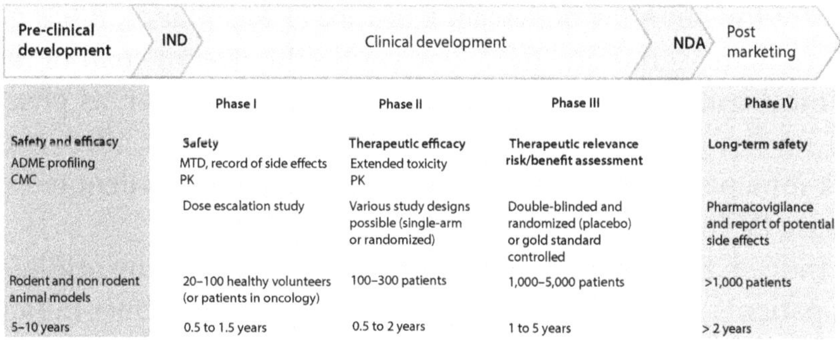

Figure 5.1 Overview of the FDA approval pipeline [7].

inducing unacceptable toxicity, which is referred to as maximum tolerated dose [3]. About the 70% of the drugs reach a level of safeness that allows them to overcome phase I [2].

However, being safe is not a satisfactory requisite for drug approval, as it has been estimated that about 10% of the drugs passing phase I trials are approved for clinics [4]. Assessing drug effectiveness is the main purpose of phase II trials, which are dedicated to groups of 100-300 patients that are affected by the disease the drug is designed for. In particular, the main goal in phase II is to define a treatment plan for the new drug, such as the administration route, the optimal dosage and the dosing interval if repeated administration is required. Phase III is employed to both confirm the findings of phase II and improve the statistical significance on a population of thousands of patients. The main goal of phase III is to prove whether or not the new drug is more effective than the standard employed for a specific disease.

Products that have overcome all the phases of human trials must be submitted to FDA as New Drug Application (NDA) for formal approval before marketing. The NDA must provide all the laboratory preclinical data on animal models, the data analyses of the clinical trials in the phases I to III, and a complete datasheet on the pharmacokinetic and manufacturing specifications of the drug. Thus, the approving agency has 60 days to accept the NDA for review and, in case of acceptance, it has no more than 10 months to review it [5]. The overall span of the clinical trials is usually from 2 to 10 years, however, as phase III involves at most few tens of thousands patients, FDA may ask for a post-marketing surveillance which is often denoted as phase IV [6].

Indeed, after marketing, a drug can be employed by millions of patients of various ethnic groups, maybe with concomitant diseases and jointly to other medications. Sometimes, under these boundary conditions, rare adverse effects arise. Indeed, clinical trials are conducted under strictly controlled conditions and patients with multiple diseases or renal dysfunctions are often discarded from the trials. On this hand, phase IV is often considered a never-ending clinical trial, since adverse reactions could be reported as long as the drug is on the market. In some few cases, drugs approved for the market have been withdrawn ensuing phase IV evaluation owing to safety issues [7].

It is worth to notice that the aforementioned discussion on FDA approval pipeline is almost identical for EMA, as far as it concerns clinical trials phase I-III [8]. There are however some technical differences among the two regulatory organs, often resulting in significant differences in the time needed for a product to arrive to the market. One important difference regards the responsibilities of the two organs; EMA is in charge to regulate the marketing of human and veterinary drugs, vaccines and other medical devices, whereas FDA is responsible also for the safety of most of U.S. food's supply and cosmetics. Another important difference is that while FDA oversees all the clinical trial phases, EMA is not responsible for the trials, whose authorization and oversight is in charge to each member states. Noteworthy, the different organization of the two agencies often results in an average of three years lag-time between US and Europe for the marketing of new drugs [9].

5.2 Nanotherapeutics

The vast majority of nanomaterials proposed for clinical translation are formulations of existing drugs in a nanosized object (nanodrugs). As already discussed in the previous chapters, the main purpose of a nanodrug is to improve the drug pharmacokinetics by increasing the circulation lifetime, which, in turn, results in higher passive accumulation at disease sites minimizing adverse effect produced by off-target distribution. In addition, nanodrugs can also alter the concentration-time profile of a drug, enabling its controlled release even in a sustained manner [10, 11]. Currently, there are 50 nanomedicines that have received clinical approval and that are available on the market [12]. Notably, most of the nanodrugs that have been approved or are under clinical investigation are composed by known chemotherapeutics. In these systems, the drug usually demonstrates either reduced side effects resulting from inherent cytotoxicity and increased water-solubility. On this regard, Doxil®, PEGylated liposomes containing doxorubicin, was the first nanodrug to receive FDA approval in 1995 for the treatment of Kaposi's sarcoma in patients affected by human immunodeficiency virus infection. Nowadays, Doxil® has not yet provided enhanced therapeutic efficacy respect to bare doxorubicin, whereas it has substantially reduced the cardiotoxicity related to the drug. To date, Doxil® use has been extended to the treatment of other diseases including ovarian cancer, and multiple myeloma [13].

Another successful liposome-encapsulated chemotherapeutic is Onivyde®. Onivyde® comprises irinotecan, a topoisomerase I inhibitor employed for the treatment of gemcitabine-resistant pancreatic tumors. It has been recently approved by both FDA and EMA as adjuvant chemotherapeutic in combination with fluorouracil and folinic acid, and is also under clinical evaluation in phase II and III for the treatment of esophagus-gastric and colorectal cancers [14]. As other liposomal formulations,

Onivyde® yielded reduced systemic toxicity in preclinical studies. However, recent investigations on the toxicity profile of liposomal irinotecan have not shown a significant safety improvement when *in vivo* compared to free irinotecan [15]. Sometimes, reduced toxicity is not a sufficient parameter to ensure the clinical translation of a nanodrug. For instance, liposome-encapsulated cisplatin such as L-NDDP, SPI-77, lipoplatin and LiPlaCis have showed reduced toxicity and similar therapeutic efficacy to cisplatin itself, resulting in the failure of their clinical translation process [16].

To avoid further rejections, novel liposomal nanodrugs that are now under clinical trials have been improved to ensure several advantages besides reducing toxicity. For instance, the specificity of PEGylated liposomes containing doxorubicin seems to be enhanced by the inclusion of antibodies towards human epidermal receptor. Due to the addition of a targeting moiety, this nanodrug held the promise to increase the therapeutic action of doxorubicin. Unfortunately, the approval process has been recently stopped by the manufacturer, as the substantial advantages over standard treatments were not confirmed [17]. An alternative approach relies on exogenous triggered release of drugs from liposomal nanodrugs. This is the case of ThermoDox®, a lysolipid thermally sensitive liposome encapsulating doxorubicin which readily undergoes conformational change upon heating to 40 °C, slightly above body's temperature, releasing the drug. The product is currently in phase III of clinical trials for the treatment of liver cancer combined with radiofrequency ablation therapy [18]. Other FDA approved nanodrugs based on liposomes that are available for clinical use include treatments for eye-related pathologies, fungal infections, postoperative sustained release of painkillers and many others, and are extensively reviewed elsewhere [19].

A pivotal role in nanomedicine is driven by polymeric NPs; the category with the highest number of clinically available nanomedicines, and the second after liposomes if considered the overall number of products under clinical investigation (Figure 5.2). Polymer nanodrugs are usually designed with the aim to be: i) degradable polymeric nanocapsules designed with similar purposes of liposomal nanodrugs, or ii) polymer–drug conjugates that have as main goal the increase of drug biocompatibility or solubility. It is worth to remember here that polymers are also extensively coupled to other classes of nanomaterials as coatings, in order to increase the overall therapeutic efficacy, as in the case of PEG coating for liposomes.

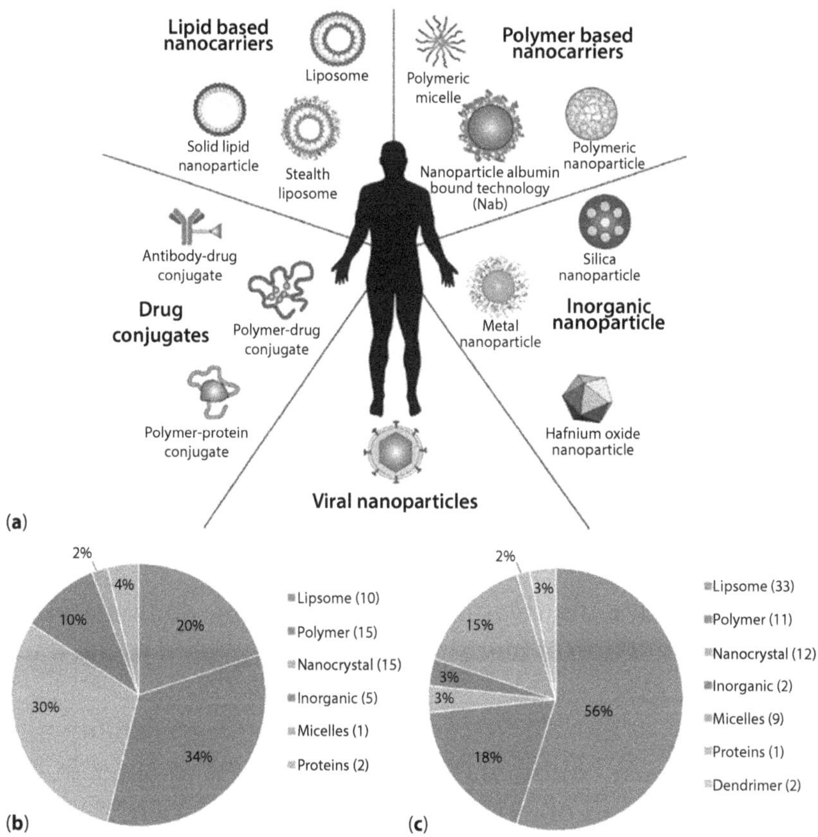

Figure 5.2 (a) Overview of the established nanomedicines either on the market or under clinical investigation. (b) Approved nanodrugs already available for clinical use and (c) nanodrugs under clinical investigations [20, 12]. (a) Reprinted with permission from [20]. (b,c) Data from [12].

One of the first FDA-approved polymeric nanodrugs was Copaxone®, an immunomodulatory drug composed by glatiramer acetate, a synthetic random polymer containing a mixture of l-glutamic acid, l-lysine, l-alanine, and l-tyrosine amino acids, which has been largely employed for the treatment of multiple sclerosis [21]. The mechanism of action of Copaxone® relies on the modulation of the innate and the adaptive immune response, promoting deviation from the pro-inflammatory to the anti-inflammatory pathways. Immune cells are stimulated to reach the diseased target undergoing inflammation event and secrete anti-inflammatory cytokines. Moreover, there are increasing evidences that Copaxone® promotes neuroprotective repairing processes, such as neurotrophic factors secretion and remyelination [22]. These benefits contributed to make Copaxone® one of the most sold drugs in U.S. in 2013 together with a PEG-conjugated formulation of filgrastim, a drug employed to alleviate chemotherapy-induced neutropenia [12]. Similarly, peginterferon beta-1a (Plegridy®), an interferon beta-1a conjugated to PEG, has recently received approval for clinical use in both EU and U.S. for the treatment of relapsing-remitting multiple sclerosis [23]. Moreover, the same nanodrug is currently investigated in preclinical studies for the assessment of anticancer properties towards melanoma xenografts established in mouse models, demonstrating notable tumor regression [24]. Other PEGylated drugs have been approved very recently for the treatment of hemophilia, demonstrating enhanced reduction of bleeding episodes compared to the standard of care [25].

Interestingly, also PLGA, owing to its biodegradability and sustained release ability, was recently approved to enter in the market. At the end of 2017 a PLGA nanoformulation of triamcinolone acetonide has been approved for the treatment of osteoarthritis knee pain with the commercial name of Zilretta®. It is a non-opioid painkiller administered as intra-articular injection which has been demonstrated to produce pain relief in patients afflicted by degenerative joint pathologies over 12 weeks.

Finally, an increasing quantity of inorganic nanomaterials including metal oxide, metal, or silica NPs, is investigated in the pre-clinical stage for therapeutic purposes. However, the only FDA-approved inorganic nanodrugs nowadays available on the market is composed by iron oxide NPs and employed for the treatment of iron deficiency anemia associated with chronic kidney disease [26]. These nanodrugs include Feraheme®, Venofer®, Ferrlecit®, Infed® and Dexferrum® which are NPs composed by an iron oxide core, coated by hydrophilic polymers that reduce their dissolution kinetics. All these nanodrugs are employed in the iron replacement therapy, as they afford the possibility of administer huge doses of NPs while minimizing the risk of iron overload in blood, thanks to the slow release profile. Noteworthy, the only metal-based nanodrug that is currently under clinical investigation is Aurimune®, which consists in gold NPs of 27 nm decorated with PEG polymer and conjugated to recombinant human tumor necrosis factor (TNF). It has been tested in clinical trials on patients with advanced or metastatic cancers that are no longer responsive to standard chemotherapy [27]. Noticeably, there are no noble metal-based nanodrugs available on the market for clinical use.

5.3 Nanodiagnostics

Compared to nanodrugs for therapeutic purposes, clinical translation of nanomaterials for diagnostic is still at its early stages. This gap is likely related to the fact that most of the non-invasive and ultrasensitive nanomaterials-enhanced diagnostic techniques rely on the use of inorganic NPs, and often on noble metal-based ones. Indeed, despite holding the great promise as revolutionary tools for detection of diseases, the only metal-based nanodiagnostic on the market are, till now, bench tools intended for clinical *in vitro* employment. For instance, colorimetric assays based on gold NPs conjugated to monoclonal anti-chorionic gonadothropin antibodies are widely employed for the detection of pregnancy states through urine analyses [28]. These tests belong to the family of lateral flow immunochromatographic assays (LFA), which, roughly, rely on the capture of the analyte from a fluid through an antigen-antibody reaction which typically leads to a color change. To date, FDA has also approved five LFA based on gold NPs for the detection of HIV [29]. Another gold NPs-based diagnostic tool called Verigene® is able to identify and quantify relevant nucleic acid sequences from biological fluids. Currently, there are two FDA-approved tests for the identification of single-nucleotide polymorphism based on the Verigene® system, and it is also employed for the detection of Gram-positive and Gram-negative bacteria and resistance determinants [30–32].

Notwithstanding the huge amount of potentially translatable nanomaterials designed for *in vivo* diagnostics, including IONPs for magnetic resonance imaging (MRI) [33], silicon-based NPs for multimodal imaging [34], carbon nanotubes for fluorescence and photoacoustic imaging (PAI [35]) and highly fluorescent quantum dots [36], currently the only nanodiagnostics that have received clinical approval is the MRI contrast agent ferumoxsil [37, 38]. Ferumoxsil, marketed in Europe as Lumirem® and in US as GastroMARK®, received FDA-approval in 1996. It consists of 400 nm siloxane-coated super paramagnetic iron oxide NPs (SPIONs), and it is routinely employed as orally administrable contrast agent for MRI examinations of the stomach and bowels [39]. Other nanosized contrast agents for MRI such as ferumoxides (Endorem® and Feridex® in Europe and US, respectively) and ferucarbotran (commercially available as Resovist®) have received approval from regulatory organs for human use. However, ferumoxides have been withdrawn from the market due to the lack of customers, and ferucarbotran is currently available only in few countries, including Japan [40, 41].

Other diagnostics that received FDA-approval and that are currently available in clinics are four contrast agents for ultrasound imaging, including three perflutren lipid microspheres and SF_6 microbubbles known as SonoVue®. However, all these contrast agents are in the micrometer size range, hence, technically, they cannot be considered as nanodiagnostics. Nevertheless, materials that exceed the nanometer range while still showing properties related to their reduced size (*e.g.* EPR effect) are considered by FDA as nanomaterials. Finally, it is worth to cite the case of ferumoxytol, which we have already mentioned among the clinically approved nanotherapeutics. It is potentially a valuable nanosized contrast agent for MRI, yet it is currently approved only for therapeutic purposes [42, 43]. Few other nanomaterials are currently in the preclinical approval phase by EMA and FDA as in vivo diagnostic tools, including the promising Cornell dots and radio-labeled NPs for PET imaging. We suggest the readers to refer elsewhere for additional details [37].

Overall, nanomaterials have remarkably revolutionized human healthcare in the last years, although nanomaterials have somehow frustrated the enormous expectations raised from the general enthusiasm that outstanding publications have generated. Following a period of general excitement in which the main purpose of researchers was to produce novel nanoplatforms comprising appealing features for just peer-review publications, nanomedicine is now going to a new era, facing up with new and exciting challenges. On the other hand, it is sometimes frustrating to notice that some scientists who have had a pivotal-role in the "golden age" are now questioning about the actual benefits nanomedicine has provided to clinics [44]. However, this field is at its early stages of development, hence it is reasonable to expect both big successes and big failures. According to a recently published work by prof. Chan, nanomedicine is probably at an evaluation stage (a turning point) in which scientists have to plan the next roadmap for future developments of nanomaterials from a practical point of view: the clinical employment [45]. Keeping in mind patient's outcome, the so called nanomedicine 2.0 could be marked by a substantial growing in the clinical translation of nanomedicines. This result can be reached only if researchers will dedicate major efforts in the quantification of nanomaterials behaviors in preclinical studies and to the validation of animal models, rather than in depicting rousing stories to persuade the audience and get their work published.

References

1. Min, Y., Caster, J. M., Eblan, M. J. & Wang, A. Z. Clinical Translation of Nanomedicine. *Chem. Rev.* 115, 11147–11190, 2015.
2. Lipsky, M. S. & Sharp, L. K. From idea to market: the drug approval process. *J. Am. Board Fam. Pract.* 14, 362–7
3. Pourgholami, M. H. *et al.* Phase I clinical trial to determine maximum tolerated dose of oral albendazole in patients with advanced cancer. *Cancer Chemother. Pharmacol.* 65, 597–605, 2010.
4. Hay, M., Thomas, D. W., Craighead, J. L., Economides, C. & Rosenthal, J. Clinical development success rates for investigational drugs. *Nat. Biotechnol.* 32, 40–51, 2014.
5. U.S. Food and Drug Administration. The FDA's Drug Review Process: Ensuring Drugs Are Safe and Effective. at <https://www.fda.gov/drugs/resourcesforyou/consumers/ucm143534.htm>
6. Suvarna V. Phase IV of Drug Development. *Perspect. Clin. Res.* 1, 57–60, 2010.
7. Ragelle, H., Danhier, F., Préat, V., Langer, R. & Anderson, D. G. Nanoparticle-based drug delivery systems: a commercial and regulatory outlook as the field matures. *Expert Opin. Drug Deliv.* 14, 851–864, 2017.
8. Van Norman, G. A. Drugs and Devices. *JACC Basic to Transl. Sci.* 1, 399–412, 2016.
9. Kramer, D. B., Xu, S. & Kesselheim, A. S. How Does Medical Device Regulation Perform in the United States and the European Union? A Systematic Review. *PLoS Med.* 9, e1001276, 2012.

10. Attama, A. A. & Umeyor, C. E. The use of solid lipid nanoparticles for sustained drug release. *Ther. Deliv.* 6, 669–684, 2015.
11. Campos, E. V. R. *et al.* Polymeric and Solid Lipid Nanoparticles for Sustained Release of Carbendazim and Tebuconazole in Agricultural Applications. *Sci. Rep.* 5, 13809, 2015.
12. Ventola, C. L. Progress in Nanomedicine: Approved and Investigational Nanodrugs Progress in Nanomedicine : 42, 742–755, 2017.
13. Barenholz, Y. (Chezy). in *Handbook of Harnessing Biomaterials in Nanomedicine* 335–398, 2012.
14. Zhang, H. Onivyde for the therapy of multiple solid tumors. *Onco. Targets. Ther.*, 9, pp. 3001–3007, 2016.
15. Kipps, E., Young, K. & Starling, N. Liposomal irinotecan in gemcitabine-refractory metastatic pancreatic cancer: efficacy, safety and place in therapy. *Ther. Adv. Med. Oncol.* 9, 159–170, 2017.
16. Caster, J. M., Patel, A. N., Zhang, T. & Wang, A. Investigational nanomedicines in 2016: a review of nanotherapeutics currently undergoing clinical trials. *Wiley Interdiscip. Rev. Nanomedicine Nanobiotechnology* 9, e1416, 2017.
17. Merrimack Pharmaceuticals, I. Merrimack Stops the Phase 2 HERMIONE Trial of MM-302 in HER2-Positive Metastatic Breast Cancer Patients. at <http://investors.merrimack.com/news-releases/news-release-details/merrimack-stops-phase-2-hermione-trial-mm-302-her2-positive>
18. Clincaltrials.gov. Phase 3 Study of ThermoDox With Radiofrequency Ablation (RFA) in Treatment of Hepatocellular Carcinoma (HCC). at <https://clinicaltrials.gov/ct2/show/NCT00617981>
19. Bulbake, U., Doppalapudi, S., Kommineni, N. & Khan, W. Liposomal Formulations in Clinical Use: An Updated Review. *Pharmaceutics* 9, 12, 2017.
20. Tran, S., DeGiovanni, P.-J., Piel, B. & Rai, P. Cancer nanomedicine: a review of recent success in drug delivery. *Clin. Transl. Med.* 6, 44, 2017.
21. Ruggieri, M., Avolio, C., Livrea, P. & Trojano, M. Glatiramer Acetate in Multiple Sclerosis: A Review. *CNS Drug Rev.* 13, 178–191, 2007.

22. Aharoni, R. Immunomodulation neuroprotection and remyelination – The fundamental therapeutic effects of glatiramer acetate: A critical review. *J. Autoimmun.* 54, 81–92, 2014.
23. Hoy, S. M. Peginterferon Beta-1a: A Review of Its Use in Patients with Relapsing-Remitting Multiple Sclerosis. *CNS Drugs* 29, 171–179, 2015.
24. Boccia, A. *et al.* Peginterferon Beta-1a Shows Antitumor Activity as a Single Agent and Enhances Efficacy of Standard of Care Cancer Therapeutics in Human Melanoma, Breast, Renal, and Colon Xenograft Models. *J. Interf. Cytokine Res.* 37, 20–31, 2017.
25. U.S. Food and Drug Administration. Food and Drug Administration. Novel drug approvals for 2017, 2017. at <www.fda.gov/drugs/developmentapprov-%0Aalprocess/druginnovation/ucm537040>
26. Bobo, D., Robinson, K. J., Islam, J., Thurecht, K. J. & Corrie, S. R. Nanoparticle-Based Medicines: A Review of FDA-Approved Materials and Clinical Trials to Date. *Pharm. Res.* 33, 2373–2387, 2016.
27. McNeil, S. E. in *Characterization of Nanoparticles Intended for Drug Delivery*. 3–8, 2011.
28. de Moraes, G. S., Cristovam, R. do A. & Savaris, R. F. Comparative analysis of the accuracy of urinary hCG tests *in vitro*. *Rev. da Assoc. Médica Bras.* English Ed. 57, 506–512, 2011.
29. Cordeiro, M., Ferreira Carlos, F., Pedrosa, P., Lopez, A. & Baptista, P. Gold Nanoparticles for Diagnostics: Advances towards Points of Care. *Diagnostics* 6, 43, 2016.
30. Wojewoda, C. M. *et al.* Evaluation of the Verigene Gram-Positive Blood Culture Nucleic Acid Test for Rapid Detection of Bacteria and Resistance Determinants. *J. Clin. Microbiol.* 51, 2072–2076, 2013.
31. Lefferts, J. A., Jannetto, P. & Tsongalis, G. J. Evaluation of the Nanosphere Verigene® System and the Verigene® F5/F2/MTHFR Nucleic Acid Tests. *Exp. Mol. Pathol.* 87, 105–108, 2009.
32. Maurice, C. B. *et al.* Comparison of assay systems for warfarin-related CYP2C9 and VKORC1 genotyping. *Clin. Chim. Acta* 411, 947–954, 2010.
33. Ling, D., Lee, N. & Hyeon, T. Chemical Synthesis and Assembly of Uniformly Sized Iron Oxide Nanoparticles for Medical Applications. *Acc. Chem. Res.* 48, 1276–1285, 2015.

34. Phillips, E. *et al.* Clinical translation of an ultrasmall inorganic optical-PET imaging nanoparticle probe. *Sci. Transl. Med.* 6, 260ra149-260ra149, 2014.
35. Gong, H., Peng, R. & Liu, Z. Carbon nanotubes for biomedical imaging: The recent advances. *Adv. Drug Deliv. Rev.* 65, 1951–1963, 2013.
36. Park, Y., Jeong, S. & Kim, S. Medically translatable quantum dots for biosensing and imaging. *J. Photochem. Photobiol. C Photochem. Rev.* 30, 51–70, 2017.
37. Park, S. M., Aalipour, A., Vermesh, O., Yu, J. H. & Gambhir, S. S. Towards clinically translatable *in vivo* nanodiagnostics. *Nat. Rev. Mater.* 2, 2017.
38. Kiessling, F., Mertens, M. E., Grimm, J. & Lammers, T. Nanoparticles for Imaging: Top or Flop? *Radiology* 273, 10–28, 2014.
39. Leung K., *Ferumoxsil. Molecular Imaging and Contrast Agent Database (MICAD).* National Center for Biotechnology Information, USA, 2004.
40. Wang, Y.-X. J. Current status of superparamagnetic iron oxide contrast agents for liver magnetic resonance imaging. *World J. Gastroenterol.* 21, 13400, 2015.
41. Wáng, Y. X. J. & Idée, J.-M. A comprehensive literatures update of clinical researches of superparamagnetic resonance iron oxide nanoparticles for magnetic resonance imaging. *Quant. Imaging Med. Surg.* 7, 88–122, 2017.
42. Varallyay, C. G. *et al.* What Does the Boxed Warning Tell Us? Safe Practice of Using Ferumoxytol as an MRI Contrast Agent. *Am. J. Neuroradiol.* 38, 1297–1302, 2017.
43. Nguyen, K.-L. *et al.* MRI with ferumoxytol: A single center experience of safety across the age spectrum. *J. Magn. Reson. Imaging* 45, 804–812, 2017.
44. Torrice, M. Does Nanomedicine Have a Delivery Problem? *ACS Cent. Sci.* 2, 434–437, 2016.
45. Chan, W. C. W. Nanomedicine 2.0. *Acc. Chem. Res.* 50, 627–632, 2017.

6

Avoiding the Persistence of Metal Nanomaterials

In the previous chapters, the physio-chemical properties of nanomaterials have been summarized (chapter 2) and their promising applications as therapeutic and diagnostic discussed (chapter 3). In chapter 4 we have comprehensively reviewed the interactions between nanomaterials and biological entities, discussing a number of issues (immune response, short blood circulation half-life, persistence in the organism) that have prevented the clinical translation of the majority of promising nanomaterials. Indeed, in chapter 5 we have overviewed the current status of nanomaterials translated to clinics, highlighting the impressive percentage of promising nanomaterials that have failed the translation to the market. In particular, most of the promising inorganic nanomaterials that have been engineered for oncology are still confined to the bench side. Noteworthy, none of the proposed noble metal-based nanomaterials have yet obtained clinical approval from FDA or EMA. It is worth to remember here that one of the key-question for FDA or EMA approbation of a novel nanomaterial is whether all of its components are completely cleared and in which time-frame; leaving residues in patients is not acceptable. Likely, the main hurdle that hampers the clinical translation of noble metals nanomaterials is related to the dilemma concerning their optimal size. Usually, noble metal NPs proposed for theranostics have a diameter over 20 nm. This size results in their fast recognition by the RES and accumulation in liver and spleen. Such persistence increases the likelihood of toxicity and the interference with common medical diagnoses. Size reduction to ultrasmall nanoparticles (USNPs) allows the efficient excretion by renal filtration but circulation half-life of USNPs is often too short for achieving efficient accumulation at target sites. Moreover, most of the physiochemical properties of metal NPs whereby they result as ideal candidates for theranostics are lost or severely altered in the ultrasmall regime. In this chapter, we will present an overview of the strategies adopted to overcome the persistence hurdles; a critical step forward toward the clinical translation of metal nanomaterials. Moreover, we will discuss a promising class of porphyrin-based nanomaterials that offer an appealing alternative to inorganic NPs as potentially clinically translatable theranostics.

6.1 Ultrasmall-in-Nano Approach

Very recently, a growing number of researchers have dedicated their efforts to engineer disassembling metal nanoplatforms able to combine theranostics features and efficient excretion of the building blocks. A ground-breaking advance in this direction relies on the ultrasmall-in-nano approach [1]. This approach consists in the design of biodegradable nanocapsules containing metal USNPs that are in the optimal size range to ensure long blood circulation and efficient uptake in the target.

The key-advances of this approach are: i) USNPs mimic the physical behavior of bigger NPs when strictly packed together, ii) the size of the nanocapsules promotes accumulation in the target and cellular uptake, and iii) the degradation products of the nanocapsules are quickly excretable or can be re-used from organisms for physiological functions.

One of the pioneering investigations on this topic was reported by Wang and co-workers in 2010. They exploited the plasmonic properties of gold USNPs to build a supramolecular aggregate mimicking optical activity of bigger NPs [2]. The system was engineered to yield good photothermal (PT) efficiency by self-assembly of three building blocks: (i) adamantane (Ad) coated 2 nm gold NPs, (ii) β-cyclodextrin –grafted polyethylenimine (CD-PEI) and (iii) Ad -functionalized PEG (Ad-PEG). The aggregates displayed remarkable stability in a wide range of temperatures at pH comprised among 4 and 10. In addition, aggregates were finely tunable in size from 40 to 118 nm by varying the stoichiometry of the three building blocks. These nanoplatforms were employed for PT therapy towards cultured cancer cells, demonstrating an enhanced heat conversion with respect to single gold USNPs. This first attempt towards a new generation of theranostics nanoplatforms was innovative, yet not devoid of issues. Two major concerns were related to the optical response of the aggregates: i) PTT was triggered by visible light, around 520 nm, strongly reducing their possible employment in clinics, and ii) their disassembling during light-triggering caused by their low stability at temperatures higher than 40 °C. In the same year another group developed independently a procedure to assemble 4.1 nm gold NPs in polymeric aggregates with a final hydrodynamic diameter of about 80 nm [3]. USNPs were assembled by employing copolymers of polylactic acid and polyethylene glycol (PLA(2K)–b-PEG(10K)–b-PLA(2K)). Compared to the aggregates produced by Wang *et al.*, this method of aggregation produced an important shift in the LSPR which displayed an interesting extinction band in the near infrared window. These aggregates demonstrated good photoacoustic (PA) contrast enhancement and, after accomplishment of the diagnostic action, biodegradation to potentially renal clearable building blocks [4].

Following these pioneering studies, similar polymer-driven approaches have been extensively adopted to develop ultrasmall-in-nano materials (Figure 6.1). For example, encapsulation of 2.2 and 5.1 nm gold USNPs coated by, respectively, glutathione or 11-mercaptoundecanoic acid was achieved by controlled aggregation of poly di(carboxylatophenoxy) phosphazene (PCPP) and methoxypoly(ethylene glycol)–block-poly(L-lysine hydrochloride) (PEG–PLL) [5]. Notably, the production of these nanomaterials is finely tunable on the size, ranging from 40 to 400 nm, and in the optical response. Indeed, the absorbance peak of these constructs is easily modulable in the 600–900 nm spectral window by varying the loading of USNPs. Notably, these nanomaterials have demonstrated both *in vitro* and *in vivo* diagnostics potential as CT and PA contrast agents, as well as *in vitro* biodegradation to harmless byproducts such as phosphate, ammonia, and 4-hydroxybenzoic acid. However, *in vivo* investigations to assess and quantify their excretion are not yet reported, reducing their potentiality. In this context, an interesting work has been published by Al-Zaki *et al.*, in which the ultrasmall-in-nano constructs were built by enveloping 1.9 nm gold USNPs with PEG-polycaprolactone micelles of 25–150 nm [6]. These composites were employed as theranostic tools exploiting their peculiar interaction with X-rays, yielding substantial CT contrast and remarkable radiotherapy enhancement. Moreover, the authors provided detailed biodistribution analyses over a three months period, reporting a noticeable accumulation of gold in the liver which halved in the following months. This result is not unexpected because the employed gold USNPs were highly hydrophobic, promoting aggregation and immune system recognition [7].

As discussed in chapter 4, renal excretion is also allowed for anisotropic nanomaterials having one dimension in the

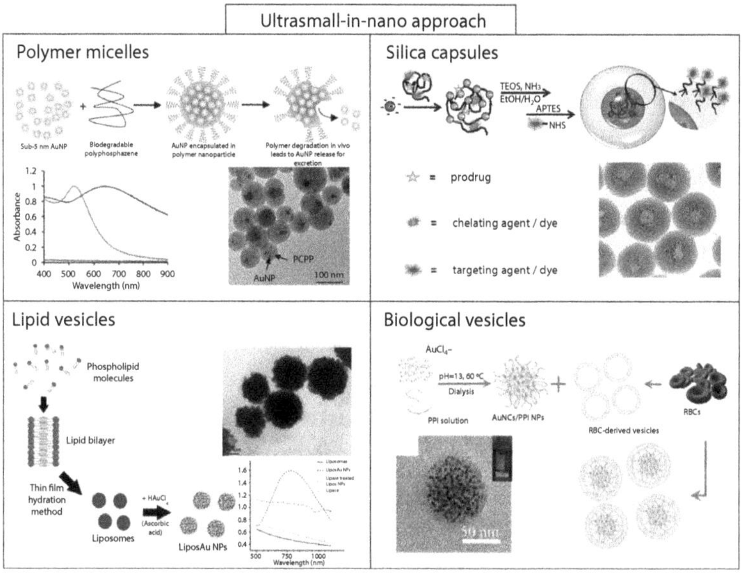

Figure 6.1 Examples of ultrasmall-in-nano constructs produced by encapsulating ultrasmall NPs in (clockwise order): polymeric micelles, silica capsules, biological vesicles (red blood cells) and lipid vesicles [5, 13, 15, 16]. (Top, left) Adapted from [5] with permission of Elsevier. (Bottom, left) Adapted with permission from [16]. Copyright 2015 American Chemical Society. (Bottom, right) Adapted with permission from [13]. Copyright 2018 American Chemical Society.

optimal size range for glomerular filtration. This is for instance the case of gold nanorods with ultrasmall diameter. Song and co-workers exploited this peculiar biological behavior to realize biodegradable nanovesicles containing gold nanorods of 8 nm in length and 2 nm in diameter [8]. Gold nanorods were held together by means of polymers (PEG and PLGA) and demonstrated a remarkable red shift of the LSPR in the NIR region. These constructs demonstrated good efficiency as PA and PET (after proper radiolabeling) contrast agents and also as therapeutic tool for enhanced PT therapy. The authors claimed for efficient renal clearance and, for this purpose, they performed some biodistribution assessments that pointed out a substantial accumulation in the RES of the injected dose. A possible explanation for the complete excretion failure might be ascribed to the reshaping of gold nanorods following laser irradiation on the LSPR [9–11]. This effect produces variations in size and shape of the nanorods, strongly decreasing their potential clearance from kidneys.

Interestingly, LSPR shift and enhanced interaction with ionizing radiation are not the only theranostics benefits arising from nanomaterials developed by the ultrasmall-in-nano approach. For instance, aggregation of fluorescent clusters greatly enhanced their luminescence through the aggregation induced emission effect (AIE) [12]. Yahia-Ammar *et al.* have reported glutathione coated gold clusters aggregated by means of the cationic polymer poly(allylamine hydrochloride) obtaining a nanoconstructs with a pH-responsive overall size ranging from 80 to 350 nm at pH 6 and 11, respectively. The aggregates were adopted for *in vitro* drug delivery with enhanced cellular uptake and improved fluorescence imaging respect to free clusters. On this regard, another very recent report has been published by Li *et al.* They have produced fluorescent gold clusters by means of plant proteins that acted as reducing agent, stabilizer and driving moieties for the self-assembly of micelles of about 100 nm [13]. The aggregates exhibited strong red fluorescence together with remarkable biocompatibility and colloidal stability and were employed for *in vivo* tumor imaging. Noteworthy, previous to mouse systemic injection, aggregates were enveloped in red blood cells to ensure prolonged blood circulation and high tumor passive uptake. Indeed, while free clusters displayed negligible blood retention and their fluorescence signal was lost by confocal fluorescence imaging only few hours after injection, red blood cells containing cluster aggregates preferentially accumulated at tumor site, and their fluorescence was well detectable 24 h after administration. AIE was also produced by the assembly of ultrasmall copper clusters in aggregates of about 20–120 nm, as recently reported by Su *et al.* Cu clusters were synthesized by employing L-cysteine as reduction and stabilizing agent, and the aggregates were produced through self-assembly of BSA-NPs conjugates at pH 3 [14].

At this pH, the assemblies showed enhanced luminescence at 620 nm, albeit being not water soluble. Their solubility was regained at pH higher than 4 or lower than 1.5 whereas their luminescence weakened. The authors did not provide stability assessment in any biological environment, hence it is hard to predict their implementation for *in vivo* applications given their dramatic alteration of solubility in response to pH variations.

Another adopted strategy for achieving USNPs agglomeration in an ultrasmall-in-nano fashion is by employing lipid vesicles. For instance, Rengan and co-workers reported the synthetic route for producing biocompatible and biodegradable 1,2-distearoyl-snglycero-3-phosphocholine/cholesterol (DSPC/CHOL) liposomes of 100–120 nm coated with gold USNPs [16]. Resembling a nanoshell geometry, these constructs showed LSPR in the NIR region, and hence were employed: i) for *in vitro* and *in vivo* PT therapy in tumor xenograft models, ii) as drug carriers in cultured cells, and iii) as CT contrast agents in phantoms. Notably, the authors performed pharmacokinetic analyses to assess the clearance capability of these nanoplatforms. They claimed for efficient clearance of the gold USNPs via hepatobiliary and renal pathways, and notably the amount of gold found in liver and kidneys was, respectively, 3% and 0.22% ID two weeks after administration.

Another appealing strategy to produce ultrasmall-in-nano constructs is by encapsulating USNPs in silica nanocapsules. This strategy provides several advantages over the other approaches, since silica is: i) biocompatible, ii) biodegradable, iii) FDA-approved as food additive, and iv) a naturally occurring compound in food and water. Moreover, silica surface is easily functionalizable with moieties of interest. In addition, degradation (hydrolysis) of non-crystalline silica NPs produces silicic acid, which is known to provide a number of health benefits [17]. One of the first report of silica nanocapsules containing USNPs was published by Hembury and co-workers, who produced nanoplatforms bearing multimodal imaging features

[18]. These constructs, named quantum rattles (QRs), consist in a hollow mesoporous silica capsule of about 150 nm containing gold NPs of mean size 7.3 nm in the cavity and gold USNPs (<2 nm) entrapped in the silica shell. While larger gold

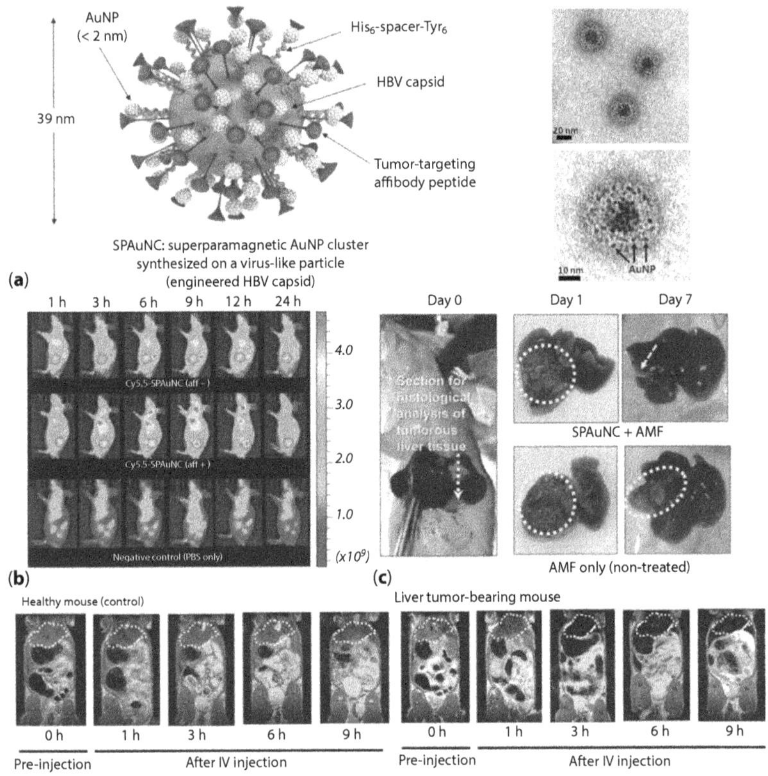

Figure 6.2 (a) Scheme of the nanoplatform composed by an engineered hepatitis B virus capsid decorated with gold USNPs and targeting moieties (left) and representative TEM images of the nanostructure at different magnifications. (b) NIR fluorescence imaging of the Cy5.5 dye-labeled nanoplatforms displaying preferential tumor accumulation (dotted red circles) when exposing targeting peptide (aff +) with respect to non-functionalized ones (aff -) and the control (PBS only). (c) Photos of cancerous livers treated with alternating magnetic field either with (top) or without (bottom) nanoplatforms injection. (d) MRI employing the nanoplatforms as contrast agent in healthy (left) and tumor-bearing mice (right) showing increased contrast in the tumor region (yellow dotted regions indicate the liver). Reprinted from [34] with permission of John Wiley & Sons Inc.

NPs confer plasmonic feature to the QRs, USNPs exhibit NIR fluorescence and paramagnetic properties that allow for three complementary imaging modalities: i) fluorescence, ii) PA imaging and iii) MRI. On the other hand, the hollow cavity allows for remarkable drug encapsulation of about 15.1% wt/wt. The authors demonstrated the theranostics efficacy of QRs in tumor bearing mice. Despite these nanoconstructs result promising, their safe translation to clinics is hampered by the presence of gold NPs whose size exceeded the glomerular filtration threshold. Our group have recently proposed an innovative route for encapsulating USNPs into biodegradable silica shells, morphologically resembling a passion fruit [15]. These nano-architectures (NAs) are composed by a polymeric core comprising functionalizable amines and plasmonic USNPs, up to 18% wt/wt [19]. USNPs are strictly packed to mimic the optical behavior of larger spherical NPs. Biodegradation of NAs to renal clearable building blocks was demonstrated in both human serum (18 hours) and in MIA PaCa-2 cancer cells (24 hours), together with their possible application as endogenous-triggered chemotherapeutics delivery platforms [20]. Interestingly, insertion of NIR dyes in the cavity of NAs yielded enhanced PA contrast, relying on fluorescence quenching of gold USNPs, which have been exploited for *ex vivo* PA imaging [21]. Moreover, the versatility of the production protocol of NAs has been recently demonstrated by the generalization to other noble metals of interests, including platinum, silver and mix of metals, and to nanostructures devoid of metals [22]. Overall, the robust, scalable and simple synthesis protocol, the extreme versatility and the biodegradation in excretable or non-toxic building blocks, make NAs one of the most promising nanoconstructs for clinical translation of noble metals., Another group has very recently reported the synthesis of ultrasmall-in-nano constructs similar to NAs, named FLASH. This nanomaterial consists in fluorescent gold nanocrystals ranging from 3 to 5 nm, embedded in a hollow silica nanocapsule of about

100 nm with a 29.6 nm shell thickness [23]. FLASH exhibited enhanced fluorescence with respect to single nanocrystals, and were effectively employed for photodynamic therapy *in vitro* against HeLa cells. However therapeutic action was achieved through irradiation with UV light, and this pose a severe limitation to clinical application and commercialization.

As discussed in chapter 2, magnetic properties of nanomaterials, such as relaxation times, change dramatically when nanoparticles are arranged in strictly packed aggregates. Combining arrays of superparamagnetic NPs with chemotherapeutics in a single nanoconstruct to achieve magnetically driven drug delivery have fostered the synthesis of diverse ultrasmall-in-nano platforms based on SPIONs. In order to produce these

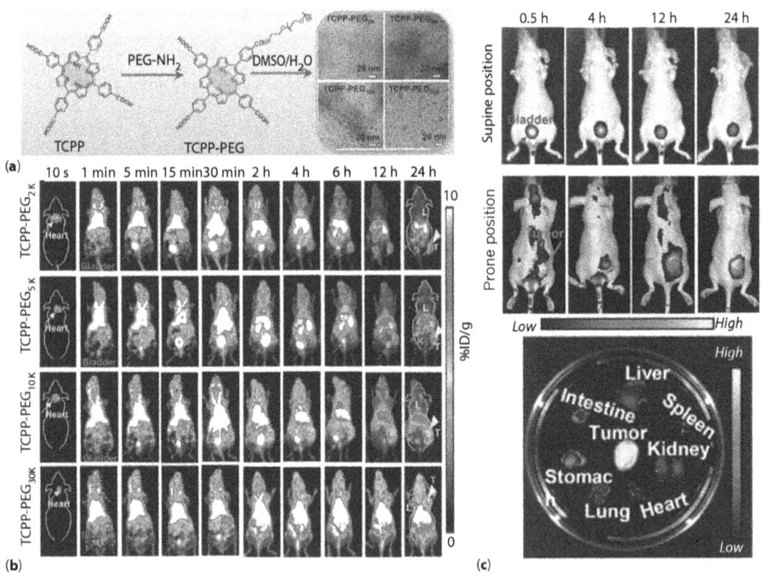

Figure 6.3 (a) Scheme of the synthesis of PEG-TCPP and TEM images of NPs synthesized with PEG of different molecular weight. (b) PET imaging of the biodistribution of PEG-TCPP over 24h in tumor-bearing mice. (c) Fluorescence imaging of PEG-TCPP during at different time steps after systemic administration in tumor-bearing mice (top) and of the explanted organs and tumor 24 h after administration (bottom) [63]. Reprinted from [63] with permission of John Wiley & Sons Inc.

nanoplatforms, many groups have exploited lipid vesicles [24, 25], silica NPs [26, 27], polymers [28–30] and even auto assemblies of SPIONs and drugs [31]. However, iron oxide NPs have shown several issues when their safety was assessed in clinical trials. A paradigmatic example is the case of Ferumoxytol, an ultrasmall SPION that initially received FDA approval in 2009 as therapeutic agent for anemia. Albeit there is an impressive amount of literature discussing its potential as MRI contrast agents, a number of adverse effects have hampered its arrival to the market as diagnostic tool. These effects include severe immune responses and anaphylactic reactions that led to patient's death in 18 cases during 5 years from drug approval [32]. These issues have forced FDA to strengthen the existing warnings to their strongest one, named *Boxed Warning* [33]. On the other hand, these concerns have stimulated researchers to look for alternative magnetic nanomaterials to be employed as MRI contrast media.

On this regard, Kwon *et al.* have recently reported an ultrasmall-in-nano theranostic tool of remarkable interest for MRI imaging and hyperthermia, that relies on the magnetic properties of gold USNPs (Figure 6.2) [34]. To synthesize these nanoplatforms, gold ions were chemisorbed and directly reduced on 36 nm hepatitis B capsids modified by a peptide with high affinity to human epidermal growth factor receptor I (EGFR), that is known to be overexpressed in many tumors [35]. Stability assessment were performed in 50% human serum solution, confirming their stability even after 12 hours. Finally, the nanoplatforms were employed in murine models, and have demonstrated an outstanding tumor targeting ability, effective MRI diagnostic and hyperthermia therapy efficacy on both subcutaneous and deep-tissue tumors. Noteworthy, biodistribution evaluation demonstrated an excellent excretion of the USNPs, as gold content in the liver decreased to 1% of the injected dose 42 days after injection. Another extremely simple approach to produce monodisperse spherical aggregates of USNPs bearing magnetic properties suitable for MRI has been recently proposed by Hou and co-workers [36]. Briefly, gold clusters exposing carboxyl groups underwent self-assembly into bigger aggregates when exposed to Gd^{3+} ions owing to ionic interactions. The formed aggregates demonstrated good luminescence intensity in the NIR region, feasibility as X-ray computed tomography (CT) and magnetic resonance imaging (MRI) contrast agents. After having assessed their biocompatibility both *in vitro* and *in*

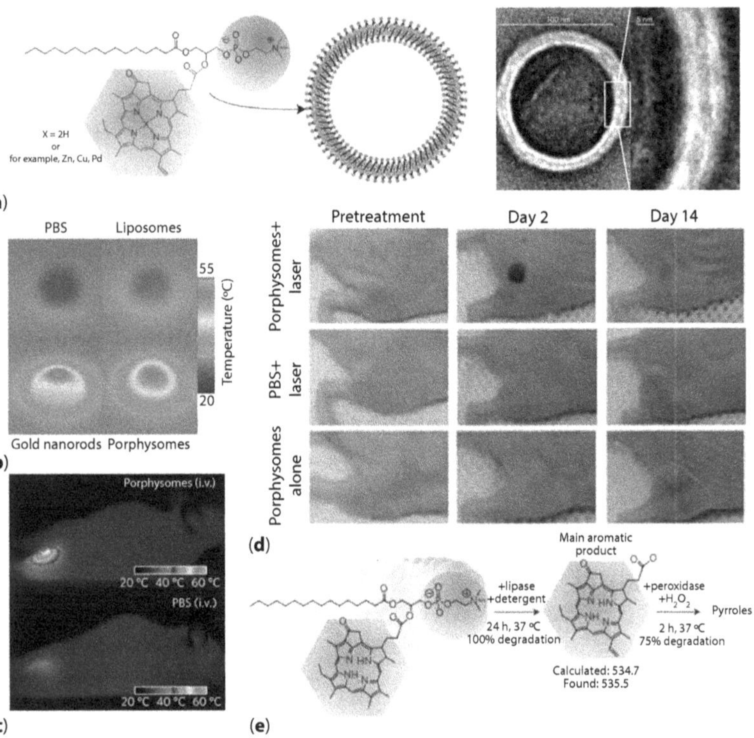

Figure 6.4 (a) Scheme of porphysome self-assembly and TEM image of the vesicle and a detail of the lipid membrane at higher magnification. (b) Photothermal efficiency benchmark of porphysomes against gold nanorods and the two controls PBS and liposomes. (c) Thermal images of tumor bearing mice injected with porphysomes or PBS 24 h prior to exposure to laser irradiation. (d) Photos of photothermal therapy efficiency on tumor bearing mice using porphysomes. (e) Scheme of the enzymatic biodegradation of porphysomes indicating the fate of each building block [68]. Reprinted with permission from [68]. Copyright 2011 Springer Nature.

vivo these nanomaterials were successfully employed as multimodal diagnostic tools in tumor-bearing mice.

6.2 Porphyrin-Based Nanomaterials

An alternative approach to conjugate excellent theranostics features avoiding metal persistence is by employing porphyrins. Porphyrins are organic compounds composed by four pyrrole subunits yielding a highly conjugated π-electron system with aromatic characters. This electronic structure is the origin of their peculiar absorption of light and of their intrinsic theranostics potentiality. A paradigmatic example is the naturally body-occurring heme group, which is a porphyrin-like molecule associated to each of the four subunits constituting hemoglobin. The aromatic π system of heme group is responsible for the intense red color of blood. Primarily, heme has a pivotal role in the oxygen transport mechanism, as each heme group chelates an iron atom that is able to bind oxygen molecules and provide precise delivery by modifying its oxidization state from Fe^{2+} to Fe^{3+} [37]. Moreover, heme group serves as endogenous contrast agent for PA imaging, owing to the different light absorption of oxygenated and deoxygenated hemoglobin [38]. Also, owing to the variation of the magnetization state in oxygenated, deoxygenated and carbon oxide-inhibited hemoglobin, heme acts as endogenous contrast agent for MRI [39, 40].

Their physical properties, together with the possibility to assemble multiple imaging modalities in a single molecule, have aroused an enormous interest in the scientific community. Indeed, porphyrins are among the most investigated molecules for biomedical applications. Several groups have reported the synthesis of novel porphyrins either *de novo* or from existing ones, thereby a huge library of synthetic procedures are currently available in literature [41, 42]. Synthetic porphyrins have been extensively investigated for clinical diagnostic imaging modalities including PAI [43, 44], MRI [45–48] and fluorescence imaging [49–51]. Furthermore, the metal-chelating ability of some porphyrins has enabled their implementation in nuclear imaging. Indeed, modified-porphyrins chelating or including ^{64}Cu, ^{67}Ga, ^{68}Ga, ^{11}C, ^{48}V or ^{18}F radioisotopes have been developed and successfully employed for positron emission tomography (PET) imaging [52–57]. Finally, one of the most extensively investigated medical application of porphyrins is in photodynamic therapy (PDT), due to the reactive oxygen species (ROS) generation following light absorption [58–61].

However, their aromatic behavior results in poor water solubility, and then in their aggregation in aqueous solution, limiting their employment in biological environment [62]. One of the strategies employed to increase the bioavailability of porphyrins is the conjugation to other moieties, *e.g.* polymers, which increase their stability in biological media. A noteworthy example in this sense has been recently published by Cheng and co-workers who synthesized porphyrins-based nanoparticles by conjugating PEG chains to meso-tetra(4-carboxyphenyl)porphyrin (TCPP) (Figure 6.3) [63]. Interestingly, the as prepared NPs are size-tunable by simply varying the molecular weight of PEG from 2 to 30 kDa, yielding NPs whose hydrodynamic diameter ranged from about 4.6 to 10.1 nm. After radiolabeling with ^{60}Cu, the TCPP-PEG NPs were administered to tumor-bearing mice to assess their biodistribution by means of PET imaging. While the smallest NPs exhibited excellent renal clearance, the biggest one provided enhanced tumor uptake due to EPR. Interestingly TCPP-PEG of intermediate size, synthesized employing PEG of 10 kDa, resulted the best compromise for medical applications. Indeed, the biodistribution evaluation by fluorescence imaging resulted in an enhanced accumulation in the tumor site and in the bladder 24 h after systemic administration.

Similarly, another group has very recently proposed the synthesis of self-assembled porphyrin NPs by conjugating poly(vinyl alcohol) (PVA) to porphyrins derivatives [64]. Briefly, PVA was conjugated to pyropheophorbide through ester formation and the conjugates underwent self-assembly into nanostructures of about 100 nm in water. Interestingly, hydrophobic drugs or dyes or other diagnostic tools can be easily encapsulated in the NPs during the self-assembly process, leading to one step production of a complete nanotheranostics. Overall, these NPs were successfully loaded with doxorubicin and radiolabeled with ^{64}Cu, yielding suitable nanoplatforms for *in vivo* PET, NIR fluorescence imaging and chemotherapeutic delivery. Moreover, pharmacokinetics investigations demonstrated their prolonged blood circulation with respect to free drug and, notably, a conspicuous decrease of heart accumulation, hence lowering the inherent cardiotoxicity of doxorubicin.

Another approach for realizing porphyrins-based NPs relies on the lipophilic attitude of porphyrins which can be then incorporated into lipid nanostructures, such as liposomes [65]. Liposome encapsulation, besides providing the well-known advantages such as enhanced blood circulation and target accumulation, also prevented porphyrins aggregation, preserving their photophysical properties [66, 67]. However, liposome encapsulation of porphyrins often relies on their insertion in the lipid membrane. This strategy poses a limit to the amount of porphyrins that can be loaded without altering colloidal stability [67]. An elegant solution to this issue was proposed in 2011 by Lovell and co-workers, who synthesized lipid-porphyrin conjugates that underwent to self-assembly into organic liposome-like nanostructures in aqueous media (Figure 6.4) [68]. These NPs, named porphysomes, overcome the loading limitation since each lipid constituting the nanostructure bear one porphyrin, resulting in an overall amount of more than 80000 porphyrins per porphysome. The morphology of these novel nanoplatforms was investigated by TEM analysis, revealing a vesicular structure of about 100 nm comprising a shell made by a bilayer of lipid-porphyrin conjugates. The structure is highly versatile as a number of porphyrins with sundry photophysical properties can be employed to tune the optical features of the final porphysomes. The authors also demonstrated that metal ions can be inserted in the lipid bilayer by simply conjugating metal-chelating porphyrins to the lipids. Another outstanding behavior of this nanomaterial is the self-quenching resulting from the packaging of a huge number of porphyrins in a nanosized volume. Owing to this effect, which was even more pronounced when porphysome were decorated with PEG, porphysomes acted as photothermal transducer with an efficiency comparable to gold nanorods. Following the demonstration of porphysome *in vivo* feasibility for PT treatment of solid tumors, as PAI contrast agent and NIR fluorescent reporter, the authors investigated the fate of porphysome, which displayed excellent biocompatibility and enzymatic biodegradability.

Following their first report, porphysomes employment has been generalized to a huge number of therapies and diagnostic imaging modalities. For instance, Jin *et al.* demonstrated that porphysomes can be used as triggered PDT agents. Indeed, by decorating porphysomes with targeting moieties for folate receptors, the self-quenching moiety was impaired and fluorescence restored only upon uptake by folate-positive cells. Localized quenching impairment in cancer cells overexpressing folate receptor enabled both *in vivo* porphysome tracking through fluorescence imaging and targeted singlet oxygen production [69]. Production of porphysomes by employing metal-binding porphyrins allowed for radio labeling with ^{64}Cu, which unlocked their nuclear imaging potential. Indeed, porphysomes were explored as PET/fluorescence dual imaging agents to guide the surgical removal of prostate tumor and the identification of bone micrometastatic tumors [70].

A noteworthy report to mention is related to the synthesis of organic-inorganic hybrid nanostructures called cerasomes, coupled with porphyrins [71]. This novel class of nanomaterials is composed by a lipid vesicular scaffold coated by a silicate layer. The strength of these nanoplatforms relies on the preserved advantages of liposomes coupled to the shielding silica layer that acts as lipid stabilizer in biological environment. In their work, Liang and coworkers produced porphyrins-conjugated cerasomes by covalently coupling silica precursors and porphyrins to multifunctional lipids. Briefly, vesicles spontaneously formed upon dispersion of lipids in aqueous media, and the silicate layer was built by standard sol-gel methods. These nanostructures afforded higher stability with respect to classical liposomal counterpart and enhanced fluorescence intensity compared to free porphyrins. Furthermore, porphyrins-conjugated cerasomes displayed excellent PDT features, as the inherent porosity of the external silica layer did not prevent the diffusion of oxygen molecules through the lipid bilayer.

Overall, porphyrin-based nanomaterials, and porphysomes in particular, have undeniably marked a paradigm shift in the way nanomedicine is conceived. The extreme versatility of porphysomes either as diagnostic or therapeutic tools, together with their non-toxicity at concentration as high as 1 g/kg and their biodegradability make them promising tools to overcome some important hurdles preventing the clinical translation of nanomaterials. On the other hand, nanomedicine could hardly waive applications of paramount importance such as enhanced/localized radiation therapy, CT diagnostic or surface-enhanced Raman scattering (SERS) which are prerogative of metal NPs. On this regard, we have comprehensively reviewed the groundbreaking topic of ultrasmall-in-nano constructs, which bypass the non-biodegradability of metal NPs, enhancing their excretion kinetics. In this direction, rather than being an organic-replacing of metal NPs, porphysomes represent a complementary tool to unlock the enormous potential of nanotheranostics, shifting them from the bench to the bedside.

References

1. Cassano, D., Pocoví-Martínez, S. & Voliani, V. Ultrasmall-in-Nano Approach: Enabling the Translation of Metal Nanomaterials to Clinics. *Bioconjug. Chem.* 17; 29(1): 4–16. 2017.

2. Wang, S. *et al.* Photothermal Effects of Supramolecularly Assembled Gold Nanoparticles for the Targeted Treatment of Cancer Cells. *Angew. Chemie Int. Ed.* 49, 3777–3781, 2010.
3. Tam, J. M. *et al.* Controlled Assembly of Biodegradable Plasmonic Nanoclusters for Near-Infrared Imaging and Therapeutic Applications. *ACS Nano* 4, 2178–2184, 2010.
4. Yoon, S. J. *et al.* Utility of biodegradable plasmonic nanoclusters in photoacoustic imaging. *Opt. Lett.* 35, 3751, 2010.
5. Cheheltani, R. *et al.* Tunable, biodegradable gold nanoparticles as contrast agents for computed tomography and photoacoustic imaging. *Biomaterials* 102, 87–97, 2016.
6. Al Zaki, A. *et al.* Gold-loaded polymeric micelles for computed tomography-guided radiation therapy treatment and radiosensitization. *ACS Nano* 8, 104–112, 2014.
7. Al Zaki, A., Hui, J. Z., Higbee, E. & Tsourkas, A. Biodistribution, Clearance, and Toxicology of Polymeric Micelles Loaded with 0.9 or 5 nm Gold Nanoparticles. *J. Biomed. Nanotechnol.* 11, 1836–46, 2015.
8. Song, J. *et al.* Ultrasmall Gold Nanorod Vesicles with Enhanced Tumor Accumulation and Fast Excretion from the Body for Cancer Therapy. *Adv. Mater.* 27, 4910–4917, 2015.
9. Harris-Birtill, D. *et al.* Gold nanorod reshaping *in vitro* and *in vivo* using a continuous wave laser. *PLoS One* 12, e0185990, 2017.
10. González-Rubio, G. *et al.* Femtosecond laser reshaping yields gold nanorods with ultranarrow surface plasmon resonances. *Science (80-.).* 358, 640–644, 2017.
11. Gordel, M. *et al.* Post-synthesis reshaping of gold nanorods using a femtosecond laser. *Phys. Chem. Chem. Phys.* 16, 71–78, 2014.
12. Yahia-Ammar, A., Sierra, D., Mérola, F., Hildebrandt, N. & Le Guével, X. Self-Assembled Gold Nanoclusters for Bright Fluorescence Imaging and Enhanced Drug Delivery. *ACS Nano* 10, 2591–2599, 2016.
13. Li, Z. *et al.* Plant Protein-Directed Synthesis of Luminescent Gold Nanocluster Hybrids for Tumor Imaging. *ACS Appl. Mater. Interfaces,* 10(1), pp 83–90, 2017.
14. Su, X. & Liu, J. pH-Guided Self-Assembly of Copper Nanoclusters with Aggregation-Induced Emission. *ACS Appl. Mater. Interfaces* 9, 3902–3910, 2017.

15. Cassano, D., Rota Martir, D., Signore, G., Piazza, V. & Voliani, V. Biodegradable hollow silica nanospheres containing gold nanoparticle arrays. *Chem. Commun.* 51, 9939–9941, 2015.
16. Rengan, A. K. *et al. In Vivo* Analysis of Biodegradable Liposome Gold Nanoparticles as Efficient Agents for Photothermal Therapy of Cancer. *Nano Lett.* 15, 842–848, 2015.
17. Martin, K. R. The chemistry of silica and its potential health benefits. *J. Nutr. Health Aging* 11, 94–7
18. Hembury, M. *et al.* Gold-silica quantum rattles for multimodal imaging and therapy. *Proc. Natl. Acad. Sci. U. S. A.* 112, 1959–64, 2015.
19. D'Apice, R. & Voliani, V. Increasing the metal loading in passion fruit-like nano-architectures. *Adv. Mater. Lett.* 8, 1156–1160, 2017.
20. Cassano, D. *et al.* Biodegradable passion fruit-like nano-architectures as carriers for cisplatin prodrug. *Part. Part. Syst. Charact.*, 2016.
21. Avigo, C., Cassano, D., Kusmic, C., Voliani, V. & Menichetti, L. Enhanced photoacoustic signal of passion fruit-like nanoarchitectures in a biological environment. *J. Phys. Chem. C* 121, 6955–6961, 2017.
22. Cassano, D., David, J., Luin, S. & Voliani, V. Passion fruit-like nano-architectures: a general synthesis route. *Sci. Rep.* 7, 43795, 2017.
23. Kim, T. *et al.* Synthesis of Fluorescent Au Nanocrystals–Silica Hybrid Nanocomposite (FLASH) with Enhanced Optical Features for Bioimaging and Photodynamic Activity. *Langmuir* 34(1), pp. 173–178, 2017.
24. Bixner, O. & Reimhult, E. Controlled magnetosomes: Embedding of magnetic nanoparticles into membranes of monodisperse lipid vesicles. *J. Colloid Interface Sci.* 466, 62–71, 2016.
25. Salvatore, A., Montis, C., Berti, D. & Baglioni, P. Multifunctional Magnetoliposomes for Sequential Controlled Release. *ACS Nano* 10, 7749–7760, 2016.
26. Huang, L. *et al.* Multifunctional magnetic silica nanotubes for MR imaging and targeted drug delivery. *Chem. Commun.* 51, 3923–3926, 2015.
27. Cano, M. & de la Cueva-Méndez, G. Self-assembly of a superparamagnetic raspberry-like silica/iron oxide nanocomposite

using epoxy–amine coupling chemistry. *Chem. Commun.* 51, 3620–3622, 2015.
28. Rocha, N. *et al.* Novel nanoaggregates with peripheric superparamagnetic iron oxide nanoparticles and organic cores through self-assembly of tailor-made block copolymers. *RSC Adv.* 4, 24428–24432, 2014.
29. Yar, Y. *et al.* Development of tailored SPION-PNIPAM nanoparticles by ATRP for dually responsive doxorubicin delivery and MR imaging. *J. Mater. Chem. B*, 6, 289–300, 2018.
30. Zhu, K., Deng, Z., Liu, G., Hu, J. & Liu, S. Photoregulated Cross-Linking of Superparamagnetic Iron Oxide Nanoparticle (SPION) Loaded Hybrid Nanovectors with Synergistic Drug Release and Magnetic Resonance (MR) Imaging Enhancement. *Macromolecules* 50, 1113–1125, 2017.
31. Jeon, H. *et al.* Poly-paclitaxel/cyclodextrin-SPION nano-assembly for magnetically guided drug delivery system. *J. Control. Release* 231, 68–76, 2016.
32. Vasanawala, S. S. *et al.* Safety and technique of ferumoxytol administration for MRI. *Magn. Reson. Med.* 75, 2107–2111, 2016.
33. U.S. Food and Drug Administration. FDA strengthens warnings and changes prescribing instructions to decrease the risk of serious allergic reactions with anemia drug Feraheme (ferumoxytol). *Drug safety communications*, 2015.
34. Kwon, K. C. *et al.* Superparamagnetic Gold Nanoparticles Synthesized on Protein Particle Scaffolds for Cancer Theragnosis. *Adv. Mater.* 29, 1701146, 2017.
35. Herbst, R. S. Review of epidermal growth factor receptor biology. *Int. J. Radiat. Oncol.* 59, S21–S26, 2004.
36. Hou, W. *et al.* Nanoparticles for multi-modality cancer diagnosis: Simple protocol for self-assembly of gold nanoclusters mediated by gadolinium ions. *Biomaterials* 120, 103–114, 2017.
37. Zhang, Y. & Lovell, J. F. Porphyrins as Theranostic Agents from Prehistoric to Modern Times. *Theranostics* 2, 905–915, 2012.
38. Wang, X., Xie, X., Ku, G., Wang, L. V. & Stoica, G. Noninvasive imaging of hemoglobin concentration and oxygenation in the rat brain using high-resolution photoacoustic tomography. *J. Biomed. Opt.* 11, 24015, 2006.

39. Pauling, L. & Coryell, C. D. The Magnetic Properties and Structure of Hemoglobin, Oxyhemoglobin and Carbonmonoxyhemoglobin. *Proc. Natl. Acad. Sci.* 22, 210–216, 1936.
40. Kwong K. The Road to fMRI Using Endogenous MR Blood Contrast. Uludag K., Ugurbil K., Berliner L. (eds) *fMRI: From Nuclear Spins to Brain Functions. Biological Magnetic Resonance*, vol 30. Springer, Boston, MA. 2015
41. Singh, S. *et al.* Synthesis and Photophysical Properties of Thioglycosylated Chlorins, Isobacteriochlorins, and Bacteriochlorins for Bioimaging and Diagnostics. *Bioconjug. Chem.* 21, 2136–2146, 2010.
42. Lindsey, J. S. Synthetic Routes to meso -Patterned Porphyrins. *Acc. Chem. Res.* 43, 300–311, 2010.
43. Luciano, M. *et al. In vivo* photoacoustic tumor tomography using a quinoline-annulated porphyrin as NIR molecular contrast agent. *Org. Biomol. Chem.* 15, 972–983, 2017.
44. Banala, S. *et al.* Quinone-fused porphyrins as contrast agents for photoacoustic imaging. *Chem. Sci.* 8, 6176–6181, 2017.
45. Haroon-Ur-Rashid, Umar, M. N., Khan, K., Anjum, M. N. & Yaseen, M. Synthesis and relaxivity measurement of porphyrin-based Magnetic Resonance Imaging (MRI) contrast agents. *J. Struct. Chem.* 55, 910–915, 2014.
46. Wu, B. *et al.* MRI-guided tumor chemo-photodynamic therapy with Gd/Pt bifunctionalized porphyrin. *Biomater. Sci.* 5, 1746–1750, 2017.
47. Jahanbin, T., Sauriat-Dorizon, H., Benderbous, S. & Korri-Youssoufi, H. Gadolinium Meso-Tetrakis(4-Pyridyl)Porphyrin as a MRI Contrast Agent: Comparison with Anionic and Cationic Metallo-Porphyrins. *J. Colloid Sci. Biotechnol.* 4, 57–63, 2015.
48. Sour, A. *et al.* Four Gadolinium(III) Complexes Appended to a Porphyrin: A Water-Soluble Molecular Theranostic Agent with Remarkable Relaxivity Suited for MRI Tracking of the Photosensitizer. *Inorg. Chem.* 55, 4545–4554, 2016.
49. Peng, Q., Soler, A. M., Warloe, T., Nesland, J. M. & Giercksky, K.-E. Selective distribution of porphyrins in skin thick basal cell carcinoma after topical application of methyl 5-aminolevulinate. *J. Photochem. Photobiol. B Biol.* 62, 140–145, 2001.

50. Hillemanns, P. *et al.* Photodetection of cervical intraepithelial neoplasia using 5-aminolevulinic acid-induced porphyrin fluorescence. *Cancer* 88, 2275–2282, 2000.
51. Cubeddu, R., Canti, G., Taroni, P. & Valentini, G. Study of porphyrin fluorescence in tissue samples of tumour-bearing mice. *J. Photochem. Photobiol. B Biol.* 29, 171–178, 1995.
52. Iwai, K., Kimura, S., Ido, T. & Iwata, R. Tumor uptake of [48V] vanadyl-chlorine e6Na as a tumor-imaging agent in tumor-bearing mice. *Int. J. Rad. Appl. Instrum. B.* 17, 775–80, 1990.
53. Fazaeli, Y. *et al.* Preparation and preliminary evaluation of [67Ga]-tetra phenyl porphyrin complexes as possible imaging agents. *J. Radioanal. Nucl. Chem.* 288, 17–24, 2011.
54. Fazaeli, Y. *et al.* Development of a 68Ga-Fluorinated Porphyrin Complex as a Possible PET Imaging Agent. *Nucl. Med. Mol. Imaging (2010).* 46, 20–26, 2012.
55. Gonçalves, N. P. F. *et al.* Synthesis and biological distribution study of a new carbon-11 labeled porphyrin for PET imaging. Photochemical and biological characterization of the non-labeled porphyrin. *J. Porphyr. Phthalocyanines* 19, 946–955, 2015.
56. Entract, G. M. *et al.* Development of PDT/PET Theranostics: Synthesis and Biological Evaluation of an 18 F-Radiolabeled Water-Soluble Porphyrin. *Mol. Pharm.* 12, 4414–4423, 2015.
57. Shi, J. *et al.* Transforming a Targeted Porphyrin Theranostic Agent into a PET Imaging Probe for Cancer. *Theranostics* 1, 363–370, 2011.
58. Pushpan, S. K. *et al.* Porphyrins in photodynamic therapy - a search for ideal photosensitizers. *Curr. Med. Chem. Anticancer. Agents* 2, 187–207, 2002.
59. Ethirajan, M., Chen, Y., Joshi, P. & Pandey, R. K. The role of porphyrin chemistry in tumor imaging and photodynamic therapy. *Chem. Soc. Rev.* 40, 340–362, 2011.
60. O'Connor, A. E., Gallagher, W. M. & Byrne, A. T. Porphyrin and Nonporphyrin Photosensitizers in Oncology: Preclinical and Clinical Advances in Photodynamic Therapy. *Photochem. Photobiol.* 85, 1053–1074, 2009.
61. Sternberg, E. D., Dolphin, D. & Brückner, C. Porphyrin-based photosensitizers for use in photodynamic therapy. *Tetrahedron* 54, 4151–4202, 1998.

62. Aveline, B. M., Hasan, T. & Redmond, R. W. The effects of aggregation, protein binding and cellular incorporation on the photophysical properties of benzoporphyrin derivative monoacid ring A (BPDMA). *J. Photochem. Photobiol. B Biol.* 30, 161–169, 1995.
63. Cheng, L. *et al.* Renal-Clearable PEGylated Porphyrin Nanoparticles for Image-Guided Photodynamic Cancer Therapy. *Adv. Funct. Mater.* 27, 1702928, 2017.
64. Luo, Y. *et al.* 'One-Pot' Fabrication of Highly Versatile and Biocompatible Poly(vinyl alcohol)-porphyrin-based Nanotheranostics. *Theranostics* 7, 3901–3914, 2017.
65. Derycke, A. S. L. & de Witte, P. A. M. Liposomes for photodynamic therapy. *Adv. Drug Deliv. Rev.* 56, 17–30, 2004.
66. Richter, A. M. *et al.* Liposomal Delivery of a Photosensitizer, Benzoporphyrin Derivative Monoacid Ring a (BPD), to Tumor Tissue in a Mouse Tumor Model. *Photochem. Photobiol.* 57, 1000–1006, 1993.
67. Huynh, E. & Zheng, G. Porphysome nanotechnology: A paradigm shift in lipid-based supramolecular structures. *Nano Today* 9, 212–222, 2014.
68. Lovell, J. F. *et al.* Porphysome nanovesicles generated by porphyrin bilayers for use as multimodal biophotonic contrast agents. *Nat. Mater.* 10, 324–332, 2011.
69. Jin, C. S., Cui, L., Wang, F., Chen, J. & Zheng, G. Targeting-Triggered Porphysome Nanostructure Disruption for Activatable Photodynamic Therapy. *Adv. Healthc. Mater.* 3, 1240–1249, 2014.
70. Liu, T. W. *et al.* Inherently multimodal nanoparticle-driven tracking and real-time delineation of orthotopic prostate tumors and micrometastases. *ACS Nano* 7, 4221–4232, 2013.
71. Liang, X., Li, X., Yue, X. & Dai, Z. Conjugation of Porphyrin to Nanohybrid Cerasomes for Photodynamic Diagnosis and Therapy of Cancer. *Angew. Chemie Int. Ed.* 50, 11622–11627, 2011.

7

Conclusions and Perspectives

Nanomaterials have demonstrated the potential to revolutionize the way in which neoplasms are diagnosed and treated. Some efficient treatments relying on organic nanomaterials are already in the market while ~~the~~ even more promising ones based on noble metals are still on the bench scale. In particular, the intrinsic features of nanomaterials offer the possibility of the development of synergistic non-invasive treatments, by designing unique theranostic agents.

Despite the giant number of proposed nanoplatforms for development of healthcare products in the last decade, almost all have led to failure before the clinical stage. This is related to lack of sufficient knowledge of the regulatory and industrial requirements by researchers and the lack of available standard regulatory frameworks [1]. The pipeline for the development of a nanomaterial for healthcare is composed by its *in silico*/*in vitro* investigations, pre-clinical and manufacturing validation, and to clinical pilot and phase II/III validations. It is worth to notice that only the most promising nanomaterials can pass ~~to~~ the costly pre-clinical and following assessments. For a better understanding on the validation steps, we would like to suggest to readers the story of the first approved nanomaterial for healthcare application, Doxil [2].

Chiefly, a nanomaterial has to work efficiently and safely to attract industrial interests. It has to meet good manufacturing practice (GMP) standards, be ready to be scalable (up to 1 kg in the pre-clinical phase), be more efficient compared to the standard of care, adhere to regulatory analytical requirements, be stable, be reproducible, be controlled (all impurities, surfactants, and other involved molecules known and quantified), be simple (the more complex is the material the higher the risks of pre-clinical failure), be flexible and transferable [1, 3]. As recently reported, also a complete set of absorption/distribution/metabolism/excretion (ADME) investigations has to be fully provided in a couple of animal models, such as mice and rabbits [4, 5]. For a complete discussion on the parameters for quality and safety evaluation of nanomaterials for biomedical applications, we suggest the readers to other recent works [1, 5–7].

Nowadays, more than 40 nanomaterials have been approved for healthcare applications (organic or metal-oxide materials), but there is still a lack of specific general protocols for their pre-clinical assessment [6, 8, 9]. Global regulatory trends are yet to be defined. As alternative, safety/toxicology for small molecules have been frequently adapted to evaluate the behaviors of nanomaterials [7, 10]. Nevertheless, the standard development program applied to small molecules cannot be applied to nanotheranostics [10]. Indeed, nanomaterials are complex 3D-constructs comprising multiple components with preferred spatial arrangements [1, 11]. Due to this complexity, there is a general agreement to allow specific regulatory framework for each new nanomaterial on a product-by-product basis [8, 12]. This is consistent with the recently published protocol of regulatory agencies [12]. This evaluation strategy is due to the various characterization methods, physicochemical properties, and biological interactions of the involved nanomaterials [12]. Nevertheless, international cooperation and harmonized strategies between regulatory agencies are desirable in order to produce standard evaluation guidelines and boost this promising and fast-growing field. Remarkably, a profound knowledge of nanomaterials and characterization methods is needed in order to avoid unpredicted effects on patients, such as potential immune reactivity [7]. It is worth to remembering here that in the nano-range, small size/shape-changes result in dramatic change of behaviours [8]. Thus, standardized quality control protocols and assays have to be developed and validated in order to effectively monitor and characterize both the physicochemical features of nanomaterials (such as size, dispersion, morphology and charge) and to assess their performance, pharmacokinetics, specific cellular uptake, interaction with immune cells and organisms [6–8].

It should be noted that strong interactions between experimental and computational scientists would be highly desirable. Indeed, such interactions could greatly enhance the predictive accuracy of the investigations and speed-up the development process.

While some organic nanomaterials have reached the agencies approbation, metal nanomaterials still demonstrate a major issue: the persistence. Persistence and accumulation in organism after the medical action is the major concern that has hampered their clinical translation. Indeed, the first concept for agencies approbation of therapeutics relies on the complete excretion of all the components of the agent after the desired action in an optimal time frame [1]. Leaving residues in patients is not acceptable [1]. In this book, besides a profound presentation of the behaviors of materials at the nanoscale and their real or promising biomedical applications, we have comprehensively discussed this key-question and the approach to unlock the features of metal nanomaterials for healthcare. Indeed, persistence is the first concept to address while developing a novel nanotheranostics, before the consideration of other concepts such as "4S parameters" (size, shape, surface properties and mechanical stiffness of nanomaterials), vascular residence, tumor accumulation and phagocytic sequestration [5, 13]. Clearance of nanomaterials from kidneys has been demonstrated to be the most practical pathway to avoid undesirable toxic effects. The possibility to employ this excretion pathway while maintaining desirable theranostic moieties is related to the design of all-in-one biodegradable nanoplatforms. The most groundbreaking advancement for their development is the recently introduced ultrasmall-in-nano approach [14]. Disassembling nanomaterials would be the key-technology to overcome the concern of safe medical-employment of noble metal nanoparticles opening new horizons in medicine, and paving the way for new paradigms in the next generation of theranostics. Despite the field is very young, personalized and effective treatments of diseases based on noble metal nanoparticles may be no longer a dream, but a real possibility in the very next future.

References

1. Eaton, M. A. W., Levy, L., and Fontaine, O. M. A. Delivering nanomedicines to patients: A practical guide. *Nanomedicine Nanotechnology, Biol. Med. 11*, 983–992, 2015.
2. Barenholz, Y. (Chezy). Doxil® — The first FDA-approved nano-drug: Lessons learned. *J. Control. Release 160*, 117–134, 2012.
3. Alkilany, A. M., and Murphy, C. J. Toxicity and cellular uptake of gold nanoparticles: what we have learned so far? *J. Nanoparticle Res. 12*, 2313–2333, 2010.
4. Dawidczyk, C. M., Kim, C., Park, J. H., Russell, L. M., Lee, K. H., Pomper, M. G., and Searson, P. C. State-of-the-art in design

rules for drug delivery platforms: Lessons learned from FDA-approved nanomedicines. *J. Control. Release 187*, 133–144, 2014.
5. Anchordoquy, T. J., Barenholz, Y., Boraschi, D., Chorny, M., Decuzzi, P., Dobrovolskaia, M. A., Farhangrazi, Z. S., Farrell, D., Gabizon, A., Ghandehari, H., Godin, B., La-Beck, N. M., Ljubimova, J., Moghimi, S. M., Pagliaro, L., Park, J.-H., Peer, D., Ruoslahti, E., Serkova, N. J., and Simberg, D. Mechanisms and Barriers in Cancer Nanomedicine: Addressing Challenges, Looking for Solutions. *ACS Nano 11*, 12–18, 2017.
6. Anselmo, A. C., and Mitragotri, S. Nanoparticles in the clinic. *Bioeng. Transl. Med. 1*, 10–29, 2016.
7. Sainz, V., Conniot, J., Matos, A. I., Peres, C., Zupanoio, E., Moura, L., Silva, L. C., Florindo, H. F., and Gaspar, R. S. Regulatory aspects on nanomedicines. *Biochem. Biophys. Res. Commun. 468*, 504–510, 2015.
8. Sandoval, B. (MacDonald). Perspectives on FDA's Regulation of Nanotechnology: Emerging Challenges and Potential Solutions. *Compr. Rev. Food Sci. Food Saf. 8*, 375–393, 2009.
9. Desai, N. Challenges in Development of Nanoparticle-Based Therapeutics. *AAPS J. 14*, 282–295, 2012.
10. Schellekens, H., Stegemann, S., Weinstein, V., de Vlieger, J. S. B., Flühmann, B., Mühlebach, S., Gaspar, R., Shah, V. P., and Crommelin, D. J. A. How to Regulate Nonbiological Complex Drugs (NBCD) and Their Follow-on Versions: Points to Consider. *AAPS J. 16*, 15–21, 2014.
11. Voliani, V., Gemmi, M., Francés-Soriano, L., González-Béjar, M., and Pérez-Prieto, J. Texture and Phase Recognition Analysis of β-NaYF 4 Nanocrystals. *J. Phys. Chem. C 118*, 11404–11408, 2014.
12. Malinoski, F. J. The nanomedicines alliance: an industry perspective on nanomedicines. *Nanomedicine Nanotechnology, Biol. Med. 10*, 1819–1820, 2014.
13. Sun, T., Zhang, Y. S., Pang, B., Hyun, D. C., Yang, M., and Xia, Y. Engineered Nanoparticles for Drug Delivery in Cancer Therapy. *Angew. Chemie Int. Ed. 53*, 12320–12364, 2014.
14. Cassano, D., Pocoví-Martínez, S., and Voliani, V. Ultrasmall-in-Nano Approach: Enabling the Translation of Metal Nanomaterials to Clinics. *Bioconjug. Chem. accepted*, 2017. acs.bioconjchem.7b00664.

Index

Lightning Source UK Ltd.
Milton Keynes UK
UKHW02n1345060718
325331UK00003B/71/P

9 781119 418276